What others are saying abo

D0114826

"Neil Miller is making a transformative contr[...] this book on vaccines — a mindful, liberating [...] to be a classic [...] the holistic health literature. Hygieia's highest recommendation to everyone who loves children and the future of our planet." —Jeannine Parvati Baker, Director, Hygieia College, Childbirth Educator, and author of *Hygieia: A Woman's Herbal, Conscious Conception,* and *Prenatal Yoga*

"Mr. Miller points out the dangers of the 'mandatory' vaccines and of several others. His descriptions of each illness and delineation of the controversy are noteworthy." —ALA Booklist

"Compelling evidence! This book deeply affected me. I strongly recommend it to all concerned parents." —Rayna Siegler-Dineen, M.A., Early Childhood Educator

"This book on vaccines should be read by every parent and every health professional. I only wish it had been available when my wife and I had to make the difficult decision of whether or not to vaccinate our daughter." —Marvin Surkin, Ph.D., Natural Health Practitioner

"I have read your book on vaccines and was deeply moved and extremely appreciative..." —Christine Ostic, Concerned Parent

"The book was a 'Mind Blower.' Thank you." —J. Stewart, New Mom

"Your book is excellent — I'm spreading the word!" —Cynthia Goldenberg, Concerned Mother, whose once healthy son is now autistic as a result of the MMR vaccine

"...there is a growing controversy on this subject and Mr. Miller needs to be heard." —George R. Schwartz, M.D., Physician, Toxicologist, and Senior Editor of *Principles and Practice of Emergency Medicine*

"Congratulations!! Finally there is something to give patients when they inquire about this overwhelming conundrum. I've already told many people about this important contribution." —Janet Zand, N.D., Doctor of Naturopathy, Oriental Medicine, and Certified Acupuncturist

"This book is a must for all who have, or are contemplating having, children." —NAPRA Trade Journal

"A growing number of people are refusing to have their children immunized. Mr. Miller believes this issue is about to explode." —The Boston Herald

"There are grounds for questioning both the safety and efficacy of current childhood vaccination programs. These reasons are reviewed with clarity and thoroughness in the main body of this book." —Harold E. Buttram, M.D.

VACCINES: ARE THEY REALLY SAFE AND EFFECTIVE?

— A Parent's Guide To Childhood Shots

By Neil Z. Miller

New Atlantean Press
Santa Fe, New Mexico

VACCINES: ARE THEY REALLY SAFE AND EFFECTIVE?
— A Parent's Guide To Childhood Shots

By Neil Z. Miller

All rights reserved. No part of this book may be reproduced, transmitted, or utilized in any form or by any means, electronic, photographic or mechanical, including photocopying, recording, or by any information storage and retrieval system, without written permission from the author, except for brief quotations in literary articles and reviews.

International Standard Book Number:
1-881217-10-8
Library of Congress Catalog Card Number:
92-81105

Copyright © 1992, 2001 by Neil Z. Miller

10th Printing... January 2001, Revised and updated
New Millennium Edition (110,000 copies in print)

Cataloging-in-Publication Data
Miller, Neil Z.
  Vaccines : are they *really* safe and effective? a parent's guide
to childhood shots / by Neil Z. Miller.
      p. cm.
  Includes bibliographical references.
  1. Vaccination of children. 2. Immunization of children—Complications
and sequelae. 3. Communicable diseases in children. I. Title
614.47—dc20   92-81105
ISBN 1-881217-10-8: $8.95 Softcover

Cover Photo: Carmen Ruiz

Printed in the United States of America

Published by:
New Atlantean Press
PO Box 9638, Santa Fe, NM 87504

Thinktwice Global Vaccine Institute:
www.thinktwice.com

TABLE OF CONTENTS

FOREWORDS
  by George R. Schwartz, MD.....7
  by Harold E. Buttram, MD.....9
PREFACE.....13
"MANDATORY" VACCINES.....17
  Polio.....17
  Diphtheria.....24
  Measles.....25
  Rubella (German Measles).....29
  Mumps.....30
  Tetanus.....31
  Pertussis (Whooping Cough).....32
MORE VACCINES.....41
  Acellular Pertussis (Japanese Whooping Cough).....41
  Hemophilus influenza type b (Hib).....42
  Conjugated Hib.....43
  Hepatitis B.....44
  Influenza (Flu).....44
  Pneumonia.....44
  Chickenpox.....45
  Smallpox.....45
LONG-TERM EFFECTS.....47
  The Immune System.....47
  Genetic Mutation.....48
  AIDS.....49
  Developmental Disabilities.....51
  Post-Vaccinal Encephalitis.....52
  Autism.....52
  Hyperactivity/Minimal Brain Damage.....54
  Violent Crime.....55
  Drug Abuse.....56
MORE VACCINE INFORMATION.....57
  The National Childhood Vaccine Injury Act.....57
  Vaccine Contraindications: High Risk Individuals.....57
  Reporting Vaccine Reactions.....58
  Promoting Vaccine Safety.....62
  Claims for Compensation.....63
  Are Vaccines Mandatory?.....64
  Natural Immunity.....67
SUMMARY and CONCLUSION.....69
NOTES.....71

*This book is dedicated
to parents and children
everywhere.*

F OREWORD

By George R. Schwartz, M.D.

I approached Neil Miller's book, *Vaccines: Are They Really Safe and Effective?*, with some trepidation, fearing a reckless diatribe against vaccination. My basic roots are in the traditional medical system, and I have advocated immunizations along the guidelines of the Centers for Disease Control (CDC). In fact, all of my children have received preventive immunizations. Yet, I have been aware of a growing movement within this country and other parts of the world toward questioning "routine" immunizations. By "routine" I mean the usual "baby shots," and not vaccines for particular high-risk groups or for special occupations or travel. Certainly the smallpox vaccine is an example of one routine shot which was eventually discontinued when the morbidity (occurrence of the illness) from the immunization exceeded the benefits.

Into this controversy and fray, Mr. Miller has elected to enter. His is a passionate and articulate voice — one which cannot be dismissed easily. He has researched the subject extensively, and while I do not agree with some of his conclusions, I recognize that a new and intelligent voice has entered the arena.

Mr. Miller has used hundreds of references and he provides his sources. Although the tone of the book is occasionally extreme, it is clear when looking at the broader picture that Mr. Miller simply wants the best for his children and for other children as well. In his book, Mr. Miller questions routine immunizations. Therefore, his references tend toward the iconoclastic rather than the supportive variety in the medical literature. But his book is not an attempt at justifying existing practices, as by design it takes a strong stance in the anti-vaccination camp.

Why then should I — a physician who basically advocates the standard vaccinations, except in specific cases where there is a medical basis for avoiding them — be writing this foreword? I believe that there is a growing controversy on the subject and Mr. Miller needs to be heard. I need not agree with all of his conclusions in order to recognize a sincere desire to inject new information (and in some cases highlight older information) into the public arena. Similarly, I see a need for those professionals who are proponents of routine immunizations to explain to a new and perhaps more questioning generation their rationale. They need to respond to Mr. Miller through forums and the media — since the debate is going on less in professional circles than in the popular press as well as on radio and television.

Mr. Miller's book, *Vaccines: Are They Really Safe and Effective?*, is a voice seeking dialogue and requiring counterpoint.

George R. Schwartz, M.D.
Physician and Toxicologist
Santa Fe, New Mexico

F OREWORD

By Harold E. Buttram, M.D.

There is at present time an ominous trend in America towards deteriorating health in children and young adults, a trend which is well substantiated by scientific statistical reports. Allergic diseases such as asthma and eczema are rapidly increasing in both frequency and severity. Autoimmune diseases (afflictions in which antibodies or immune cells attack the tissues of one's own body) have increased manyfold in the past several generations. Perhaps most ominous of all is the rise in childhood behavioral disorders, including hyperactivity and learning disorders, with approximately 15 percent of children now being classified as learning disabled. A substantial portion of today's children are receiving frequent courses of antibiotics for treatment of recurrent ear infections and/or respiratory illness, a pattern which suggests an increasing prevalence of immune impairment when compared with earlier generations. Among young adults of today there are the newly emerging and poorly understood syndromes of chemical sensitivity and chronic fatigue, conditions which are disabling millions of our youth who should be entering the prime of their lives.

Unquestionably there are multiple causes for these adverse health trends. Unhealthful dietary patterns and exposures to toxic environmental chemicals certainly play major roles. However, our concern here is to the possible role that the routine mass inoculation of children may be playing in the increasing patterns of disabled immunity. There is one question which must be addressed: Do vaccination programs stunt or in any way thwart the normal development of the immune systems of children? As admirably reviewed in the present monograph, there are sound grounds for believing that the answer may be in the affirmative. Basing his statements on scientific literature, the author shows that the incidence of many common infections had already been declining as a result of improved sanitation before introduction of vaccines, and that this decline was barely accelerated, if at all, by the vaccines. He also shows that there may be a direct relationship between vaccinations and the modern epidemics of chronic fatigue, autoimmune disorders, AIDS, learning disabilities, and other health problems as well.

In order to better understand the concerns noted above, it would be well to review the development of the immune system following birth. The newborn infant comes into the world with a relatively undeveloped immune system. The infant does carry antibodies from its mother which persist for about 6 months, but the lymph nodes are small and rudimentary, the plasma cells are sparse in the bone marrow and lymph nodes, and immunoglobulin synthesis is low. Normally, soon after birth, the infant begins to respond to multiple antigenic stimuli from bacterial flora which rapidly populate his skin, upper respiratory tract, and bowel, as well as the microbial and parasitic infections (estimated at one every 6 weeks) acquired from the environment. This immunologic experience is reflected in progressive hyperplasia of the lymph follicles, a gradual increase in plasma cells, and an increase in immunoglobulin synthesis. In other words, the immature immune system must run a gauntlet of infectious challenges in order to become strong and resistant, a process which under normal circumstances requires 10 to 12 years.

In former times the so-called minor childhood diseases of measles, mumps, and rubella (German measles) may have served a major role in the normal development and strengthening of the immune systems of children. By altering this former pattern with vaccinations, have we set the stage for the serious chronic diseases now occurring with increasing frequency? Once again, has the overall effect been that of stunting the development of the immune systems of children? There are good reasons for believing that this is the case.

On December 1, 1988, the New York Times published an article on findings by Dr. John Walker-Smith of St. Bartholomew's Hospital in London, an expert on intestinal diseases of children. In this article Dr. Walker-Smith reported on a sharp increase in Crohn's disease (affecting the small intestines) in children of East Indian origin *who had grown up in Great Britain*, while in India the disease is "very, very rare indeed." Dr. Walker-Smith believes that the decline of many childhood infections might allow children in the West to grow up without the vigorous development of their immune system defenses that such infections would ordinarily promote.

Additional evidence in support of this hypothesis is found in a report from Afghanistan entitled, "The Adverse Effects of Antipyretics in Measles," by A. S. Ahmady and A. R. Samadi (*Indian Pediatrics,* January 1981, pp. 49-52). In this report it was found that those children with measles who were treated with antipyretics, such as aspirin or Tylenol, to lower fever and inhibit the typical skin rash had significantly prolonged duration of illness and increased incidence of respiratory complications and diarrhea. The remarkable discovery was made that children with the most violent, highly febrile form of the disease and marked skin rash actually had the best prognosis for recovery. Although the authors were cautious in drawing conclusions, it could be inferred that interference with the natural course of the disease significantly dampened the immune responses of the children. If this is true, it may be assumed that the measles vaccine, and possibly others as well, may have a comparable effect.

For these reasons and those reviewed with clarity and thoroughness in the main body of this book, there are grounds for questioning both the safety and efficacy of current childhood vaccination programs. The time is long overdue for a complete reassessment of these procedures. As in all things dealing with human affairs, science thrives best in an atmosphere of freedom. Mandated childhood vaccinations being the antithesis of freedom, the effects of continuing with these programs will be to freeze and crystallize the advances of science in this area. Admittedly, a full review of current procedures will take time, since the legitimate advances of science usually move slowly. In the meantime, as advised by the author, every parent should be allowed full freedom to accept or reject vaccines for their children. They should be allowed the privilege of "informed consent," the same as with any medical procedure that includes the possibility of adverse reactions.

Harold E. Buttram, M.D.
Family Practice
Quakertown, Pennsylvania

"Who shall [make our decisions], when doctors disagree?"
—Alexander Pope, in *Moral Essays*

P REFACE

This book came about as a result of my search to find the truth behind vaccines. When my son was born the matter became important to me. I began by gathering stacks of information from local, state, college, and medical libraries. Much of this information was taken directly from scientific journals. One by one I studied each "mandatory" vaccine. What were the symptoms of the disease it was meant to protect against? If the disease were contracted, how dangerous could it be? I also looked for 1) solid proof that the vaccine was responsible for a general decline in the incidence of the disease, 2) evidence that the vaccine is effective (Does it offer true immunity?), and 3) side effects and safety.

Slowly, the pieces of the puzzle began to fall into place. Many of the vaccines could not show that they were responsible for a decline in the incidence of the disease. Some of the graphs in this book portray this fact by showing that many of these diseases were declining in number and severity on their own, *before* the vaccines were introduced. Many of the vaccines also failed to show evidence of their ability to confer immunity. In fact, some studies show that the disease is more likely to be contracted by those who are vaccinated against it than by those who are left alone. Finally, many of the vaccines are unsafe. Thousands of children have been damaged by them. Seizures, retardation and death are only a few of the many potential "side-effects."

In spite of these findings, I was even more shocked to learn that many powerful individuals within the organized medical profession — the Medical-Industrial Complex — including influential members of the World Health Organization (WHO), the American Medical Association (AMA), the American Academy of Pediatrics (AAP), the Federal Centers for Disease Control (CDC), the Food and Drug Administration (FDA), major medical journals, hospitals, health professors, scientists, coroners, and the vaccine manufacturers, are aware of much of this information as well, but appear to have an implicit agreement to obscure the facts, minimize the truth, and deceive the public. For years — ever since the early part of this century when the organized medical profession was granted a legal monopoly on health care — it has stifled dissenting individuals within and outside of the profession from making their warnings known. But doctors are merely human; their united front is only a stoic facade that hides their many differences and concerns. For example, some doctors do warn parents about the potential dangers associated with vaccines. A few even require parents to sign a form absolving the doctor from liability if the child is damaged from the shots. Medical experts who refuse to inoculate their own children are also making a powerful statement. So are the medical policy-makers who cower to business concerns, or who elect to disregard pertinent data, especially when a whole nation is willing to trust their partial conclusions while placing their children into their care.

On the other hand, few parents are prepared to arrive at their own conclusions regarding the vaccine decision. They tenaciously, almost religiously, trust their doctors and pediatricians. They are afraid to ask questions, or to even consider all of their options. Many parents are simply unwilling to take responsibility for health-related decisions. But parents are ultimately responsible for their own health and the health of their children.

I wrote this book (and two additional books on this subject as well — turn to pages 79 and 80 for more information) so that parents like yourself may make a more informed decision regarding vaccines. I do not advocate them, nor do I presume to know what is best for you and your family. I merely try to present the facts in a clear and straightforward manner. Therefore, if after reading this book you still have questions and concerns, I suggest that you study the references in the back of this book, in addition to any other pertinent information you can find. In fact, I recommend that you continue with your search for the truth for as long as it takes to arrive at a proper solution to the vaccine dilemma.

Note: In an earlier draft of this book I included two personal and highly emotional accounts from anguished parents describing how a particular vaccine damaged their child. Some critics voiced disapproval at this practice, claiming an appeal to the emotions has no place in a fact-finding search. However, as I already stated in this preface, the truth has been obscured for too long. I don't see anything wrong with permitting my readers to *feel* their pain. In fact, I hope you become as outraged as I am. Real children are being damaged and dying, and real parents are having to cope with their disabilities and deaths.

Because the wounded children are often forgotten in the midst of the history and politics of this issue, these personal accounts will remain. In fact, I have added several slightly less emotional case histories (in the section on Reporting Vaccine Reactions). Many show a tendency of doctors to deny the existence of adverse events.

ACKNOWLEDGEMENTS

I wish to acknowledge the following authors and organizations for their brave and pioneering accomplishments regarding vaccines. Some of their discoveries are cited throughout the text: Hannah Allen, Harold E. Buttram, Harris L. Coulter, Barbara Loe Fisher, Walene James, Eleanor McBean, Robert S. Mendelsohn, Richard Moskowitz, Mothering (magazine), the National Vaccine Information Center, and many others too numerous to name. For all of our children, thank you.

WARNING!

The decision of whether or not to vaccinate is a personal one. The author is not a health practitioner and makes no claims in this regard. Nor does the author recommend for or against vaccines. All of the information in this book is taken from other sources and documented in the Notes section. If you have any questions, doubts, or concerns regarding any of the information in this book, go to the original source. Then research this topic even further so that you can make a wise and informed choice.

May God bless you for seeking the truth, for taking personal responsibility for your decisions, and for wanting only the very best that this world has to offer for your innocent and trusting children.

Neil Z. Miller

"It is a serious disease to worry over what has not occurred."
—Ibn Gabirol

"MANDATORY" VACCINES

Vaccines are injections that contain weakened amounts of the disease germ that they are meant to protect against. They are said to work by stimulating the body to produce antibodies — proteins that defend the body from an invasion by harmful germs.

The term "vaccine" is derived from "vacca," the Latin word for cow. This is because the material of cowpox (a disease affecting the udders of cows), was injected into people to protect them against an attack of smallpox.[1]

The idea of vaccinations to prevent disease dates back to 1796. In that year Edward Jenner, a British physician, noted that dairymaids who had caught cowpox (a minor disease), could not catch smallpox (a fatal disease). Jenner then took diseased matter from the hand of Sarah Nelmes, a local dairymaid who had become infected with cowpox, and inserted this matter into the cut arm of James Phipps, a healthy eight-year-old boy. The boy then caught cowpox. Forty-eight days later Jenner injected smallpox matter into the boy. It had no effect. This was the first recorded vaccination.[2]

Today, several vaccines exist. They are prevalent — even mandatory — in many countries. Most people trust them to be safe and effective. But, findings on seven of the more commonly administered vaccines — for poliomyelitis (polio), diphtheria, measles, German measles (rubella), mumps, tetanus, and pertussis (whooping cough) — do not support this conclusion.

POLIO

Polio is a contagious disease caused by an intestinal virus that may attack nerve cells of the brain and spinal cord. Symptoms include fever, headache, sore throat, and vomiting. Some victims develop neurological complications, including stiffness of the neck and back, weak muscles, pain in the joints, and paralysis of one or more limbs or respiratory muscles. In severe cases it may be fatal, due to respiratory paralysis.

Treatment consists of putting the patient to bed and allowing the affected limbs to be completely relaxed. If breathing is affected, a respirator or iron lung may be used. Two to three years of physiotherapy may be required.

In 1955 Dr. Jonas Salk, an American physician and microbiologist, developed a killed-virus vaccine against polio. In 1959 Dr. Albert Sabin, also an American physician and microbiologist, developed a live-virus (oral) vaccine against polio. Both vaccines are considered safe and effective in preventing polio (and the spread of the polio virus).

Findings: Many people mistakenly believe that anyone who contracts polio either becomes partially paralyzed or dies. However, in most infections caused by polio there are few distinctive symptoms.[3] In fact, the natural polio virus produces no symptoms at all in over 90 percent of the people who are exposed to it, even under epidemic conditions.[4] This has lead more than one scientific researcher to conclude that the small percentage of people who do develop paralytic polio may be "anatomically susceptible" to the disease. The vast remainder of the population may be naturally immune to the polio germ.[5]

Polio is virtually nonexistent in the United States today; however, there is no credible scientific evidence that the vaccine caused polio to disappear.[6] From 1923 to 1953, *before* the Salk killed-virus vaccine was introduced, the polio death rate in the United States and England had already declined on its own by 47 percent and 55 percent, respectively. Statistics show a similar decline in other European countries as well (Figure 1).[7] And when the vaccine did become available, many European countries questioned its effectiveness and refused to systematically inoculate their citizens. Yet, polio epidemics also ended in these countries.[8]

The number of reported cases of polio *following* mass inoculations with the killed-virus vaccine was significantly greater than *before* mass inoculations, and may have more than doubled in the U.S. as a whole. For example, Vermont reported 15 cases of polio during the one-year report period ending August 30, 1954 (before mass inoculations), compared to 55 cases of polio during the one-year period ending August 30, 1955 (after mass inoculations) — a 266% increase. Rhode Island reported 22 cases during the before inoculations period as compared to 122 cases during the after inoculations period — a 454% increase. In New Hampshire the figures were 38-129; in Connecticut they were 144-276; and in Massachusetts they were 273-2027 — a whopping 642% increase (Figure 2).[9]

Note: Doctors and scientists on the staff of the National Institute of Health during the 1950's were well aware that the Salk vaccine was ineffective and deadly. Some frankly stated that it was

Figure 1:

The POLIO DEATH RATE WAS DECREASING ON ITS OWN *BEFORE* the VACCINE WAS INTRODUCED

(Figures are from 1923 to 1953)

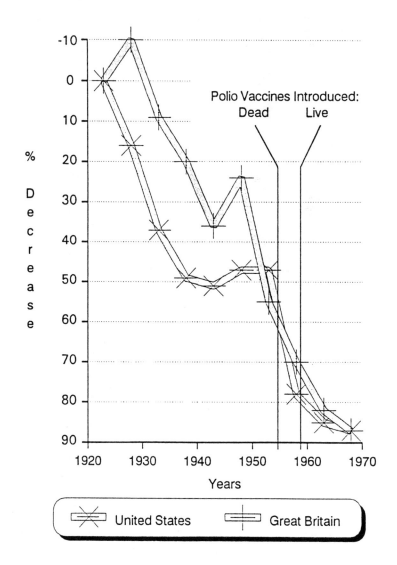

Figure 2:

CASES of POLIO *INCREASED* AFTER MASS INOCULATIONS

(Figures are for Five New England States
during 1954 and 1955)

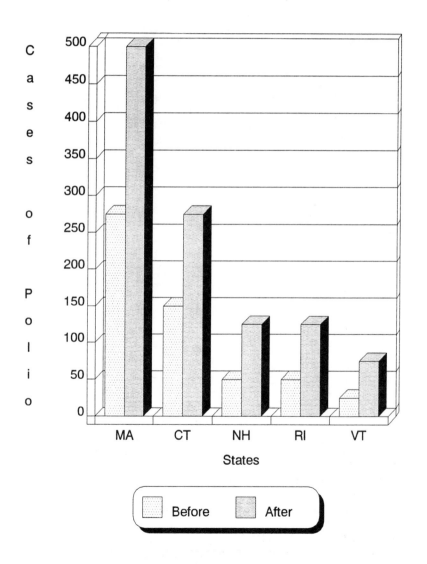

"worthless as a preventive and dangerous to take."[10] They refused to vaccinate their own children. Even Dr. Salk himself was quoted as saying: "When you inoculate children with a polio vaccine you don't sleep well for two or three weeks."[11] But the National Foundation for Infantile Paralysis, and pharmaceutical companies with a large investment in the vaccine (i.e., Parke-Davis), coerced the U.S. Public Health Service into signing a false proclamation claiming the vaccine was safe and 100 percent effective.[12]

The standards for defining polio were changed when the live-virus polio vaccine was introduced. For example, the new definition of a "polio epidemic" required more cases to be reported (35 per 100,000 instead of the customary 20 per 100,000). At this time paralytic polio was redefined as well, making it more difficult to confirm, and therefore tally, cases. Prior to the introduction of the vaccine the patient only had to exhibit paralytic symptoms for 24 hours. Laboratory confirmation and tests to determine residual (prolonged) paralysis were not required. The new definition required the patient to exhibit paralytic symptoms for at least 60 days, and residual paralysis had to be confirmed twice during the course of the disease. Finally, after the vaccine was introduced cases of aseptic meningitis (an infectious disease often difficult to distinguish from polio) were more often reported as a separate disease from polio. But such cases were counted as polio *before* the vaccine was introduced. The vaccine's reported effectiveness was therefore skewed (Figure 3).[13,14]

Note: The practice of redefining a disease when it is contracted by an "immunized" person is not new. This was a common tactic during the smallpox epidemics as well. For example, in 1936 in Great Britain the Ministry of Health admitted that the vaccine status of the individual is a guiding factor in diagnosis. In other words, if a person who is vaccinated contracts the disease, the disease is simply recorded under a different name.[15]

In 1976, Dr. Jonas Salk, creator of the killed-virus vaccine used throughout the 1950's, testified that the live-virus vaccine (used almost exclusively in the United States since the early 1960's) was "the principle if not sole cause" of all reported polio cases in the United States since 1961.[16] (The virus remains in the throat for one to two weeks and in the feces for up to two months. Thus, vaccine recipients are at risk, and are potentially contagious, as long as fecal excretion continues.)[17]

The Federal Centers for Disease Control (CDC) recently admitted that the live-virus vaccine has become the dominant cause of polio in the United States today.[18] In fact, according to CDC figures, 87 percent of all cases of polio in the United States

Figure 3:

CASES OF POLIO
WERE MORE OFTEN REPORTED
as ASEPTIC MENINGITIS
AFTER the VACCINE
WAS INTRODUCED

(Figures are from the Los Angeles County Health Index:
Morbidity and Mortality, Reportable Diseases)

Sample Months	Reported Cases of Polio	Reported Cases of Aseptic Meningitis
July 1955 (Before the oral polio vaccine was introduced):	273	50
Sept. 1966 (After the oral polio vaccine was introduced):	5	256

between 1973 and 1983 (excluding imported cases) were caused by the vaccine (Figure 4).[19] More recently, *every case of polio* in the U.S. since 1979 (excluding five imported cases) was caused by the vaccine. (And three of the five people who caught polio during foreign travel were previously vaccinated against the disease.)[20]

In Finland, where the killed-virus vaccine is used, there were *no* reported cases of polio between 1964 and 1983. However, in 1984 several Finns contracted polio thus renewing the authorities' debate on the relative effectiveness of either vaccine.[21]

Diet: In 1948, during the height of the polio epidemics, Dr. Benjamin Sandler, a nutritional expert at the Oteen Veterans' Hospital, detailed a relationship between polio and an excessive consumption of sugars and starches. He compiled records showing that countries with the highest per capita consumption of sugar had the greatest incidence of polio. He claimed that such "foods" dehydrate the cells and leech calcium from the nerves, muscles, bones, and teeth. A serious calcium deficiency precedes polio.[22]

Figure 4:

87% of ALL POLIO CASES WERE *CAUSED* by the POLIO VACCINE

CDC Figures (USA): 1973-1983

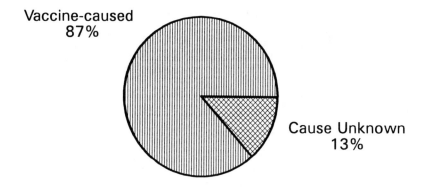

Vaccine-caused
87%

Cause Unknown
13%

Researchers have always known that polio strikes with its greatest intensity during the hot summer months. Dr. Sandler observed that children consume greater amounts of ice cream, soda pop, and artificially sweetened products in hot weather. In 1949, before the polio season began, he warned the residents of North Carolina (thorough the newspapers and radio) to decrease their consumption of these products. During that summer North Carolinians reduced their intake of sugar by 90 percent and polio decreased in that state in 1949 by the same amount. (The North Carolina State Health Department reported 2,498 cases of polio in 1948 and 229 in 1949).[23,24]

Note: One manufacturer shipped one million less gallons of ice cream during the first week alone following the publication of Dr. Sandler's anti-polio diet. Coca Cola sales were down as well. But the powerful Rockefeller Milk Trust, which sold frozen products to North Carolinians, combined forces with the Coca Cola power merchants and convinced the people that Sandler's findings were a myth and the polio figures a fluke. By the summer of 1950 sales were back to ordinary levels and polio cases returned to "normal" during that year.[25]

DIPHTHERIA

Diphtheria is a contagious disease of the upper respiratory system caused by a bacterium. Symptoms include a sore throat, fever, and swelling of the lymph nodes in the neck. As the disease progresses, a thick membrane forms on the surface of the tonsils and throat, and may extend into the windpipe and lungs. This membrane may interfere with breathing and swallowing. In severe cases this membrane can completely block the breathing passages. Other complications include heart muscle inflammation and paralysis of muscles in the throat and eyes, and of those used in breathing. Paralysis of the breathing muscles can be fatal.

Diphtheria is commonly treated with antibiotics. Complete bed rest and adequate nourishment (by infusion or nasal catheter if swallowing is possible) are equally essential.

The disease is generally conveyed by direct contact with the diphtheria germ. Thus, diphtheria is readily controlled through careful attention to simple sanitary measures.[26]

Findings: Cases of diphtheria are rare. Only four cases were reported in the United States in 1992.[27] However, a significant decline in diphtheria began long before the vaccine was discovered. In the United States, from 1900 to 1930, years before the diphtheria vaccine was introduced, a greater than 90 percent decline in reported deaths from diphtheria had already occurred.[28] Some researchers attribute this decline to increased nutritional and sanitary awareness.[29,30]

Germany began compulsory diphtheria vaccinations in 1939. After that country was thoroughly vaccinated cases of the disease skyrocketed to 150,000.[31] France initially rejected diphtheria vaccinations because of the disasters she witnessed in other countries due to its use. But after the German occupation, France was forced into submitting to the shots. By 1943, cases of diphtheria in that country had soared to nearly 47,000.[32] At the same time in nearby Norway, which refused vaccinations, there were only 50 cases.[33]

In a 1975 official report on diphtheria, the Bureau of Biologics and the FDA concluded that diphtheria toxoid "is not as effective an immunizing agent as might be anticipated." They admitted that diphtheria may occur in vaccinated individuals, and note that "the permanence of immunity induced by the toxoid...is open to question."[34]

About 50 percent of all people who contract the disease have been fully vaccinated. For example, in a 1969 outbreak in Chicago, the Board of Health reported that 37.5 percent of the cases had been fully vaccinated or showed medical evidence of full immunity. A report on another outbreak revealed that 61 percent of the total cases and 33 percent of the fatal cases had been fully vaccinated.[35]

MEASLES

Measles is a contagious disease caused by a virus that affects the respiratory system, skin, and eyes. Symptoms include a high fever (up to 105 degrees), cough, runny nose, sore, red, and sensitive eyes. Small pink spots with gray-white centers develop inside the mouth. Itchy pink spots break out on the face and spread over the body.

Approximately one in 100,000 cases lead to subacute sclerosing panencephalitis (SSPE), which causes hardening of the brain and is invariably fatal.[36] In populations newly exposed to the measles virus, serious complications among adolescents and young adults increase, thus raising mortality rates.[37] However, most cases of measles are not serious,[38] especially when large numbers of the population have been exposed to the germ.[39] Symptoms usually disappear after one to two weeks.[40]

Treatment mainly consists of allowing the disease to run its course.[41]

Before the 1960's most children in the U.S. caught measles. In 1963 a team of scientists headed by American researcher John F. Enders created a measles vaccine. Mass inoculations soon followed.

Findings: A significant decline in measles began long before the vaccine was introduced. In the United States and England, from 1915 to 1958, a greater than 95 percent decline in the measles death rate had already occurred (Figure 5).[42]

In 1900 there were 13.3 measles deaths per 100,000 population. By 1955, eight years *before* the first measles shot, the death rate had declined 97.7 percent to .03 deaths per 100,000.[43] In fact, the death rate from measles in the mid-1970's (post-vaccine) remained exactly the same as in the early 1960's (pre-vaccine).[44]

Scientists do not know how long immunity from the measles vaccine lasts.[45] According to a study conducted by the World Health Organization (WHO), chances are about 14 times greater that measles will be contracted by those vaccinated against the disease than by those who are left alone.[46] According to Dr. Atkinson of the CDC, "measles transmission has been clearly documented among vaccinated persons. In some large outbreaks... over 95 percent of

Figure 5:

The MEASLES DEATH RATE DECREASED by MORE THAN 95% *BEFORE* the VACCINE WAS INTRODUCED

(Figures are from 1915 to 1958)

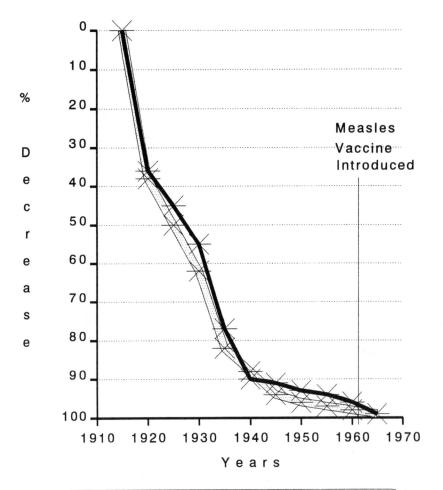

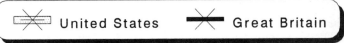

cases have a history of vaccination..."[47] Of all reported cases of measles in the U.S. in 1984, more than 58 percent of the school-age children were "adequately" vaccinated (Figure 6).[48] And in 1985, the federal government reported 1,984 non-preventable cases of measles. But 80 percent of these so-called "non-preventable" cases occurred in people who had been properly vaccinated.[49] More recent outbreaks continue to occur throughout the country, sometimes among 100 percent vaccinated populations.[50]

The measles vaccine may cause learning disability, retardation, aseptic meningitis, seizure disorders, paralysis, and death. Other researchers have investigated it as a possible cause of or co-factor for multiple sclerosis, Reye's syndrome, Guillain-Barre, blood clotting disorders, and juvenile-onset diabetes.[51] A 1995 study in *Lancet* found a link between this vaccine and bowel disease.[52]

Since the start of measles vaccinations, the peak incidence of measles no longer occurs in children, but in adolescents and young adults. The risk of pneumonia and liver abnormalities is greater in this age group. According to a recent study, such complications have increased by three percent and 20 percent, respectively.[53]

The vaccine is not recommended to children younger than 15 months, yet children of this age are most at risk from the complications of measles.[54]

Before the vaccine was introduced, it was extremely rare for an infant to contract measles. However, by 1993 more than 25 percent of all measles cases were occurring in babies under a year of age. CDC officials admit this situation is likely to get worse, and attribute it to the growing number of mothers who were vaccinated during the 1960's, '70's, and '80's. (When natural immunity is denied, measles protection cannot be passed on to their babies.)[55]

<u>Diet:</u> The *New England Journal of Medicine* recently published an article indicating that giving vitamin A to children with measles reduces the likelihood of complications and their chances of dying.[56]

The following excerpt is from a statement made by one mother testifying before the *Subcommittee on Health and the Environment,* regarding vaccine injury compensation:

"My name is Wendy Scholl. I reside in the state of Florida with my husband, Gary, and three daughters, Stacy, Holly, and Jackie. Let me stress that all three of our daughters were born healthy, normal babies. I am here to tell of Stacy's reaction to the measles vaccine...where according to the medical profession, anything within 7 to 10 days after the vaccine to do with neurological sequelae or seizures or brain damage fits a measles reaction...

Figure 6:

58% of ALL MEASLES CASES WERE CONTRACTED by PEOPLE WHO WERE VACCINATED AGAINST the DISEASE

(Figures are for all school-age children in the USA who contracted measles in 1984)

Vaccinated Prior to Contracting Measles
58%

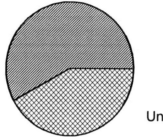

Unvaccinated
42%

"At 16 months old, Stacy received her measles shot. She was a happy, healthy, normal baby, typical, curious, playful until the 10th day after her shot when I walked into her room to find her laying in her crib, flat on her stomach, her head twisted to one side. Her eyes were glassy and affixed.

"She was panting, struggling to breathe. Her small head lay in a pool of blood that hung from her mouth. It was a terrifying sight, yet at that point I didn't realize that my happy, bouncing baby was never to be the same again.

"When we arrived at the emergency room, Stacy's temperature was 107 degrees. The first 4 days of Stacy's hospital stay she battled for life. She was in a coma and had kidney failure. Her lungs filled with fluid and she had ongoing seizures.

"Her diagnosis was 'post-vaccinal encephalitis' and her prognosis was grave. She was paralyzed on her left side, prone to seizures, had visual problems. However, we were told by doctors we were extremely lucky. I didn't feel lucky.

"We were horrified that this vaccine which was given only to ensure that she would have a safer childhood, almost killed her. I didn't know that the possibility of this type of reaction even existed. But now, it is our reality."[57]

RUBELLA

Rubella is a contagious disease which is usually so mild it often escapes detection. Symptoms include a runny nose, sore throat, and slight fever (rarely above 100 degrees). Pink, slightly raised spots appear on the face, trunk and limbs. Lymph nodes on the back of the head, behind the ears, and on the side of the neck may become tender.

Rubella is a nonthreatening disease when contracted by children. Symptoms rarely last more than two to three days. However, if a pregnant woman develops the disease during her first trimester, her baby may be born with birth defects. These include impaired vision and hearing, limb defects, mental retardation, and heart malformations.

Treatment mainly consists of allowing the disease to run its course. It is not necessary to protect children from this harmless disease.[58]

Findings: Research has demonstrated that approximately 25 percent of those vaccinated against rubella show no evidence of immunity within five years following their rubella shots.[59] In one study by Dr. Stanley Plotkin, professor of Pediatrics at the University of Pennsylvania School of Medicine, 36 percent of adolescent females who had been vaccinated against rubella lacked serological proof of immunity.[60] In a Casper, Wyoming rubella epidemic, 91 of the 125 cases (73 percent) occurred in vaccinated children.[61] In another study by Dr. Beverley Allan of the Austin Hospital in Melbourne, Australia, 80 percent of all army recruits who had been vaccinated against rubella just four months earlier still contracted the disease.[62]

Rubella is a harmless disease in childhood, and it confers natural immunity to those who contract it so they are unlikely to experience a recurrence as adults. Today, because rubella vaccinations are routinely given to children, most women never acquire natural immunity. If their vaccine-induced immunity wears off, the threat of contracting rubella during their childbearing years should actually increase.[63]

Before rubella vaccinations, nearly 85 percent of the population was naturally immune to the disease.[64] A recent survey of sixth graders in a well-vaccinated urban community revealed that about 15 percent of this group was still susceptible to rubella.[65]

In two separate scientific studies, the new rubella vaccine introduced in 1979 was found to be the cause of Chronic Fatigue Syndrome (also known as the Epstein-Barr Virus, or the "Yuppie" disease), an immunological disorder first reported in the U.S. in 1982. Given to children, the vaccine can linger in their systems for years and can be passed to adults through casual contact.[66,67]

Other adverse reactions to the rubella vaccine include arthritis, arthralgia (painful joints), and polyneuritis (pain, numbness, or paralysis in the peripheral nerves).[68] Among teenage girls, the rate of side effects is five percent to 10 percent. Among women it is greater than 30 percent.[69]

The following excerpt is from a 23 year-old woman describing her reaction to the rubella vaccine (and possibly others as well):

"On August 7, 1989 I had Rubella, Measles, and Varicella Zoster Titre IGG vaccines (for chicken pox). I am a nursing student. Within three weeks I began feeling weak, tired, and sluggish. This lead to numbness in both hands and feet. By November I developed Guillain-Barre syndrome and was hospitalized for two months. I was unable to walk, had difficulty moving my upper extremities, suffered urinary and abdominal problems, partial facial paralysis, and I lost a substantial amount of weight. Previously, I was an active healthy woman eager to finish my nursing program. My doctors do not know how I developed this syndrome."[70]

In some hospitals all employees, except physicians, are required to receive the rubella vaccine.[71] This may be because doctors are the least likely of all hospital personnel to submit to these shots. In one study published in the *Journal of the American Medical Association,* 90 percent of the obstetricians and more than two-thirds of the pediatricians refused to take the rubella vaccine. The authors of the article concluded that they were afraid of "unforeseen vaccine reactions."[72]

MUMPS

Mumps is a contagious disease caused by a virus that attacks the salivary glands. Symptoms include painful swelling beneath the ear(s) along the jaw line, fever, headache, muscle aches, and vomiting. Testicles, ovaries, and female breasts may also become inflamed and swollen.

Mumps is rarely serious, and symptoms usually disappear

within 10 days. However, approximately 35 percent of males past the age of puberty who contract mumps develop orchitis, or inflammation of the testes.[73]

Treatment mainly consists of allowing the disease to run its course. However, bed rest, a soft diet with plenty of liquids, and ice packs to reduce the swelling are often recommended.

Findings: Mumps is rarely harmful in childhood, and almost always confers lifelong immunity. Artificial immunity conferred by the mumps vaccine does not last. Recent studies show "substantial numbers of cases" of mumps among persons previously vaccinated against the disease.[74] And children vaccinated against mumps at 15 months (the recommended age), who escape the disease in childhood, are likely to suffer more serious consequences if they contract it as adolescents or young adults (because complications from mumps are more likely, and more serious, after puberty.)[75]

Orchitis, the most likely complication from mumps, rarely affects both testicles. Thus, sterility, a condition commonly linked to orchitis, is very unlikely.[76]

Adverse reactions to the mumps vaccine include rashes, itching, bruises, febrile seizures, unilateral nerve deafness, and, in rare cases, encephalitis.[77] But, a new mumps vaccine may be responsible for a recent increase in mumps-vaccine-induced encephalitis.[78]

TETANUS

Tetanus is a disorder of the nervous system caused by spores that are trapped in improperly cleaned wounds. Symptoms include depression, headaches, tightening of the body muscles, spasms of the jaw muscles (making it difficult for victims to open their mouths), and convulsions. The death rate of untreated cases has been estimated at higher than 50 percent. However, with proper treatment up to 80 percent of all cases will recover.[79]

For many years tetanus was thought to be caused by rusty nails, or from wounds that occur where manure is present. However, neither condition guarantees the disease. Although tetanus germs are more likely to grow in deep puncture wounds (due to the anaerobic conditions required for the spores to germinate), careful attention to wound hygiene will eliminate the possibility of tetanus in most cases. Wounds should be thoroughly cleaned and not allowed to close until healing has occurred beneath the surface of the skin.[80] In addition to the tetanus vaccine, tetanus toxoid, a heat-killed product of the tetanus toxin, is available. It may be given as a booster at the time of injury. Tetanus antitoxin is also available.

Findings: Among military personnel, the incidence of tetanus declined from 205 cases per 100,000 wounds (during the Civil War) to .44 cases per 100,000 wounds (during World War II) — a 99.8 percent reduction.[81] However, this disease was steadily disappearing from the developing countries long before the vaccine was introduced. Some researchers attribute this decline to an increased attention to wound hygiene.[82]

During World War II, 12 cases of tetanus were recorded; four of these cases (33 percent) occurred in military personnel who were "adequately" vaccinated.[83]

There is no credible scientific evidence indicating how often tetanus boosters are required or whether they are required at all.[84] In fact, government statistics show that until the last few years, 40 percent of the child population was not protected. Yet, infection rates from tetanus continued to decline.[85]

In order to decrease severe reactions to the tetanus vaccine, it has been significantly diluted, causing it to be clinically ineffective.[86,87] Nevertheless, complications that have occurred following tetanus vaccinations include: high fever, pain, recurrent abscess formation, inner ear nerve damage, demyelinating neuropathy (a degenerative condition of the nervous system), anaphylactic shock, and loss of consciousness.[88]

Some doctors report that tetanus toxoid does not protect and has a high mortality rate.[89]

The *New England Journal of Medicine* recently published a study showing that tetanus booster vaccinations cause T-lymphocyte blood count ratios to temporarily drop below normal. The greatest decrease occurred up to two weeks later. The report noted that these altered ratios are similar to those found in victims of acquired immune deficiency syndrome (AIDS).[90] Even a brief suppression of normal T-lymphocyte ratios is undesirable, and may be the underlying cause of at least one immunological disorder (transient hypogammaglobulinemia) found in infants.[91]

PERTUSSIS

Pertussis is a contagious disease caused by a bacterium that affects the respiratory system. Sometimes called whooping cough, this disease got its name from the high-pitched whooping noise victims make when they try to catch their breath after severe coughing attacks. Symptoms progress through three stages. In the first stage, which usually lasts one to two weeks, victims have trouble breathing, and may develop a cough and/or fever. In the second stage, which usually lasts two to three weeks, severe coughing attacks occur during the night, and then later during the day and night. The attacks can lead to inadequate oxygen circulation, which can cause convulsions. During this stage death can occur. In the final stage, coughing lessens and recovery begins. Full recovery may take two to three months.

The disease is rarely fatal.[92] However, when infants (under six months) contract pertussis, it can be serious and life-threatening.

There is no specific treatment for pertussis.[93] Antibiotics and cough suppressants have been used, but with little effect, and are generally not recommended.

A vaccine against pertussis has been available in the United States since 1936 (and was put into general use during the 1940's).

Findings: The incidence and severity of whooping cough had begun to decline long before the pertussis vaccine was introduced.[94] From 1900 to 1935, in the United States and England, *before* the pertussis vaccine was introduced, the death rate from pertussis had already declined by 79 percent and 82 percent, respectively (Figure 7).[95]

Some studies indicate that the pertussis vaccine may be only 40 to 45 percent effective.[96] Further evidence suggests that immunity is not sustained. Susceptibility to pertussis 12 years after full vaccination may be as high as 95 percent.[97] For example, during a ten month period in 1984, the state of Washington reported 162 cases; there were no deaths, no cases of brain damage, and 49 percent of the cases aged 3 months to 6 years had been fully vaccinated against the disease.[98] In fact, during that same year 2,187 nationwide cases of pertussis were reported to the CDC. Of the 560 patients aged seven months to six years with known vaccination status, 46 percent had received vaccine protection (Figure 8).[99] In 1986, in Kansas, 1300 cases of pertussis were reported. Of the patients whose vaccination status was known, 90 percent were "adequately" vaccinated.[100] And in 1993, during a pertussis outbreak in Ohio, 82 percent of younger children stricken with the disease had received regular doses of the vaccine.[101]

The diphtheria, tetanus, and pertussis vaccines are generally combined into a single formula (DPT). Both the diphtheria and tetanus vaccines are "stabilized" using formaldehyde — a known carcinogen. Each dose of DPT also contains thimerosal — a derivative of mercury — and aluminum phosphate. Mercury and aluminum are toxic to humans.[102]

Figure 7:

The PERTUSSIS DEATH RATE DECREASED by MORE THAN 75% *BEFORE* the VACCINE WAS INTRODUCED

(Figures are from 1900 to 1935)

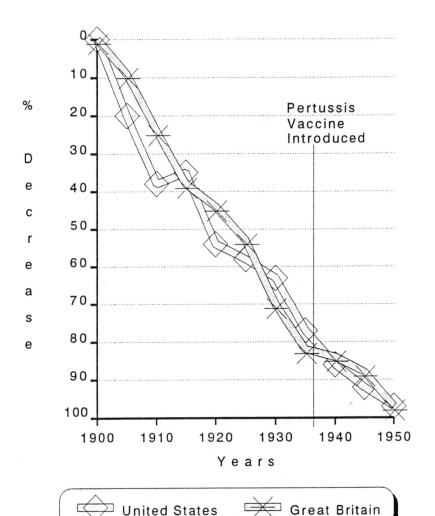

Figure 8:

46% of ALL PERTUSSIS CASES WERE CONTRACTED by PEOPLE WHO WERE VACCINATED AGAINST the DISEASE

(Figures are for all children in the USA
between the ages of 7 months and 6 years
who contracted pertussis in 1984)

Vaccinated Prior to Contracting Pertussis
46%

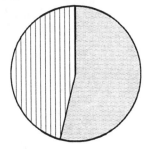

Unvaccinated
54%

The pertussis vaccine is used in animal experiments to help produce anaphylactic shock, and to cause an acute autoimmune encephalomyelitis (allergic encephalitis).[103] Post-vaccinal encephalitis may be the greatest cause of developmental and learning disabilities in the country today.[104] (See the section on Long-Term Effects.)

The United States never conducted its own clinical tests to determine whether the pertussis vaccine is safe and effective. Instead, it relies on data collected by Great Britain during the 1950's on children between six months and one-and-a-half years of age. Even though 42 of these children had convulsions within 28 days, 80 percent of the babies were 14 months of age or older, and the tests were designed to measure the efficacy (not safety) of the vaccine, U.S. health authorities use these results as evidence that the vaccine is safe to give to babies as young as six weeks of age. In fact, a two month old baby weighing less than ten pounds receives the same dose of the pertussis vaccine as a fifty pound child entering preschool.[105]

Scientists have developed an indirect test to determine the efficacy and safety of the pertussis vaccine. If the vaccine renders immunity in mice, it is considered effective in children. If the mice do not lose weight, it is presumed to be nontoxic.[106]

The pertussis vaccine may cause fever as high as 106 degrees, pain, swelling, diarrhea, projectile vomiting, excessive sleepiness, high-pitched screaming (not unlike the so-called cri encephalique, or encephalitic scream associated with central nervous system damage), inconsolable crying bouts, seizures, convulsions, collapse, shock, breathing problems, brain damage, and sudden infant death syndrome (SIDS).[107] In one study, serious reactions (including grand mal epilepsy and encephalopathy) were shown to be as high as one in 600.[108] In another study it was reported that out of 15,752 shots that were administered to children, only 18 serious reactions (shock-collapse or convulsions) occurred (1 in 875). However, each child in the study received three to five shots. Thus, approximately one out of every 200 children who received the full DPT series suffered severe reactions.[109]

A 1994 study found that children diagnosed with asthma were five times more likely than not to have received pertussis vaccine.[110] Another study found that babies die at a rate eight times greater than normal within three days after getting a DPT shot.[111] The three primary doses of DPT are given at two months, four months, and six months. About 85 percent of SIDS cases occur at one through six months, with the peak incidence at age two to four months.[112]

In a recent scientific study of SIDS, episodes of apnea (cessation of breathing) and hypopnea (abnormally shallow breathing) were measured before and after DPT vaccinations. *Cotwatch* (a precise breathing monitor) was used, and the computer printouts it generated (in integrals of the "weighted apnea-hypopnea density" — WAHD) were analyzed. The data clearly shows that vaccination caused an extraordinary increase in episodes where breathing either nearly ceased or stopped completely. These episodes continued for months following vaccinations. Dr. Viera Scheibnerova, the author of the study, concluded that "vaccination is the single most prevalent and most preventable cause of infant deaths" (Figure 9).[113]

In another study of 103 children who died of SIDS, Dr. William Torch, of the University of Nevada School of Medicine at Reno, found that more than two-thirds had been vaccinated with DPT prior to death. Of these, 6.5 percent died within 12 hours of vaccination; 13 percent within 24 hours; 26 percent within three days; and 37, 61, and 70 percent within one, two, and three weeks, respectively (Figure 10). He also found that SIDS frequencies

Figure 9:

PERTUSSIS VACCINE and STRESS-INDUCED BREATHING PATTERNS

(Summary: 17 day record of one child's breathing patterns
before and after receiving the pertussis vaccine. Values above
1000 indicate acute stress-induced breathing.)

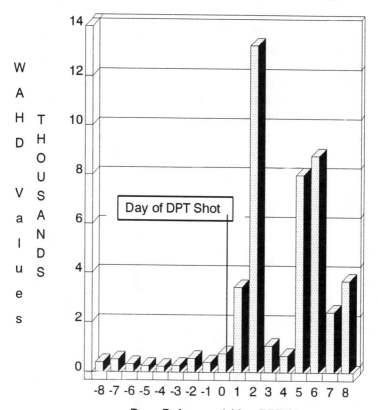

Days Before and After DPT Shot

have a bimodal peak occurrence at two and four months — the
same ages when initial doses of DPT are administered to infants.[114]

The following excerpt is from a statement made by a dis-
traught grandmother testifying before the *Committee on Labor and
Human Resources*, again regarding vaccine injury compensation:

Figure 10:

PERTUSSIS VACCINE and SUDDEN INFANT DEATH SYNDROME (SIDS)

(A Correlation Study)

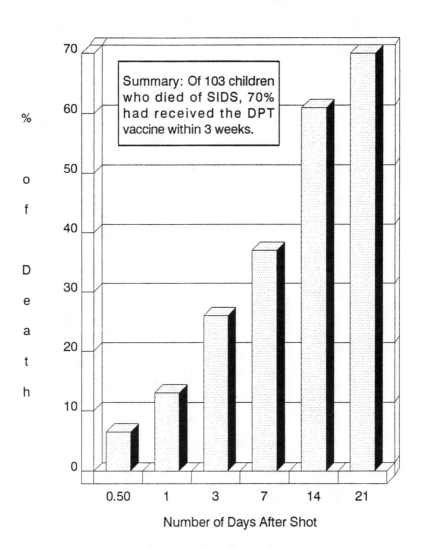

Summary: Of 103 children who died of SIDS, 70% had received the DPT vaccine within 3 weeks.

Number of Days After Shot

"My name is Donna Gary. I am a constituent of Senator Kennedy's from Massachusetts.

"Our family should have celebrated our very first granddaughter's first birthday last month. Instead, we will commemorate the anniversary of her death at the end of this month.

"Our granddaughter, Lee Ann, was just 8 weeks old when her mother took her to the doctor for her routine checkup. That included, of course, her first DPT inoculation and oral polio vaccine.

"In all her entire 8 weeks of life this lovable, extremely alert baby had never produced such a blood-curdling scream as she did at the moment the shot was given. Neither had her mother ever before seen her back arch as it did while she screamed. She was inconsolable. Even her daddy could not understand Lee Ann's uncharacteristic screaming and crying.

"Four hours later Lee Ann was dead. 'Crib death,' the doctor said — 'SIDS.' 'Could it be connected to the shot?' her parents implored.' 'No.' 'But she just had her first DPT shot this afternoon. Could there possibly be any connection to it?' 'No, no connection at all,' the emergency room doctor said definitely.

"My husband and I hurried to the hospital the following morning after Lee Ann's death to talk with the pathologist before the autopsy. We wanted to make sure he was alerted to her DPT inoculation such a short time before her death — just in case there was something else he could look for to make the connection. He was unavailable to talk with us. We waited two-and-a-half hours. Finally, we got to talk to another doctor after the autopsy had been completed. He said it was 'SIDS.'

"In the months before Lee Ann was born I regularly checked with a friend as to the state of her grandchild's condition. He is nearly a year-and-a-half older than Lee Ann. On his first DPT shot he passed out cold for 15 minutes, right in the pediatrician's office. 'Normal reaction for some children,' the pediatrician reassured. The parents were scared, but they knew what a fine doctor they had. They trusted his judgment.

"When it was time for the second shot they asked 'Are you sure it's all right? Is it really necessary?'

"Their pediatrician again reassured them. He told them how awful it was to experience, as he had, one of his infant patient's bout with whooping cough. That baby had died.

"They gave him his second DPT shot that day. He became brain-damaged.

"This past week I had an opportunity to read through printed copies of the hearings of this committee. I am dismayed to learn that this same talk has been going on for years, and nothing has seemed to progress to incorporate what seems so obvious and necessary to keep from destroying any more babies, and to compensate financially those who have already been damaged for life.

"How accurate are our statistics on adverse reactions to vaccines when parents have been told, are still being told, 'No connection to the shot, no connection at all?'

"What about the mother I have recently talked with who has a 4-year-old brain-damaged son? On all three of his DPT shots he had a convulsion in the presence of the pediatrician. 'No connection,' the pediatrician assured.

"I talked with a father in a town adjoining ours whose son died at the age of 9 weeks, several months before our own granddaughter's death. It was the day after his DPT inoculation. 'SIDS' is the statement on the death certificate.

"Are the statistics that the medical world loves to quote to say, 'There is no connection,' really accurate, or are they based on poor diagnoses, poor recordkeeping?

"What is being done to provide a safer vaccine? Who is overseeing? Will it be the same scientists and doctors who have been overseeing in the past? How much longer does the public have to wait? How are physicians and clinics going to be held accountable to see that parents are informed of the possible reactions? And how are those children who should not receive the vaccine to be identified before they are damaged — or dead?

"Today is the National Day of Prayer. My prayer is that this committee be instrumental in doing what needs to be done — and soon. May there not be yet another year pass by with more children afflicted, and some dead, because those who can do so refuse to 'make the right connection.'"[115]

Note: Despite innumerable cases like this, Senator Kennedy and his colleagues recently introduced new legislation that would attempt to vaccinate all children in the United States while severely limiting exemptions parents could claim. These bills also seek to set up a nationwide vaccine registry to track parents who resist.[116]

Mﾞ ORE VACCINES

The "mandatory" vaccines previously covered represent just a few of the many that already exist or are in the developmental stages. For example, medical scientists are working on vaccines against cancer, AIDS, venereal disease, venoms, environmental toxins, diarrhea, and even the common cold. Scientists are also experimenting with a vaccine against pregnancy, vaccines crossbred into our food supply, and a time-released "supervaccine" containing drug serum extracted from numerous remote diseases.[117]

If the principles behind the theory of vaccinations are flawed, future vaccines are probably doomed to failure as well. For example, according to Richard Moskowitz, MD, the people that need an AIDS vaccine the most are already "seriously immunocompromised." Giving a suppressive vaccine to everyone would increase the odds of developing AIDS for those already at high risk and it would weaken the general population as well.[118,119] (For an alternative view on the principles behind the theory of vaccinations, see the Germ Theory on page 66.)

Several other vaccines that already exist are introduced below.

Acellular Pertussis (Japanese Pertussis): In 1981 Japan began giving their children a new pertussis vaccine. They claim it is less toxic and more effective than the current vaccine still used in the U.S. Some authorities in this country agree, but claim that the additional cost to produce the vaccine, and the logistics involved, do not justify making the switch. However, on April 15, 1992, the AAP recommended this vaccine for the 4th and 5th doses only.[120]

The Japanese do not begin pertussis vaccinations on their children until they are two years of age. They began this practice in 1975, six years before the new pertussis vaccine was introduced. A significant drop in serious reactions following shots was immediately noticed. In the U.S. pertussis vaccinations are begun at two months, and are continued throughout the infant's early, and high-risk, months. Thus it is difficult to ascertain whether the Japanese vaccine is truly safer.[121]

In 1988 the United States tested the acellular pertussis vaccine on Swedish children. Efficacy with a two dose regimen was 69 percent. Five children died during the study. Ironically, U.S. health officials (who appear indifferent to pursuing alternatives to our imperfect whole-cell vaccine) played coy by calling for more research into the deaths, even though they occurred up to five months after vaccination, causes included heroin intoxication, and Swedish officials concluded they were unrelated to the vaccinations. Deaths that occur within hours or days of a whole-cell vaccination in the U.S. are quickly dismissed and rarely investigated.[122]

In a recent study published by the _Journal of the American Medical Association,_ two acellular pertussis vaccines were shown to be less effective than expected, and were responsible for four deaths among the tested infants.[123] And in 1987, sixty-six Japanese victims of the shots won huge awards from their government. The court recognized that the damaged plaintiffs were victimized so that the "public interest in preventing contagious diseases" wouldn't be undermined.[124]

Hemophilus influenza type b (Hib): Hemophilus influenza (no relation to the flu) is a bacterial disease that has been known to cause upper respiratory and ear infections, inflamed sinuses, pneumonia, epiglottitis (swelling of the throat that may interfere with breathing), and meningitis (inflammation of the membranes covering the brain and spinal cord). It occurs most often in Eskimo, Native American, and Negro children.[125]

In April of 1985 the Hib vaccine was approved for general use in the U.S. and was quickly recommended for all children two years old or older. (It has no efficacy in children younger than 18 months and uncertain efficacy in children 18 to 23 months old.)[126] But the peak attack period is between six months and one year, and 75 percent of all cases occur before the age of two years.[127]

The Hib vaccine is often referred to as the "meningitis" or "spinal meningitis" vaccine, but these terms are misleading. The Hib vaccine was only designed to offer some protection against the Hib bacteria, but meningitis has several causes (like the pneumococcus and meningococcus germs, and some viruses).[128] Conversely, the Hib germ may also cause upper respiratory infections, ear infections, and sinusitis, but the vaccine is not effective against these conditions.[129]

In a preliminary study conducted by the Centers for Disease Control (CDC), comprising six areas of the United States, the Hib vaccine showed an overall efficacy rate of 41 percent (for all children within the recommended two to five year old age group).[130]

However, published reports on the vaccine's effectiveness often show significantly higher percentages because members of the Medical-Industrial Complex attempted to skew the results by excluding areas where their findings didn't agree with the conclusions they sought.[131,132] For example, children who received the Hib vaccine in Minnesota were found to be five times *more likely* to contract the disease than children who did not receive the vaccine.[133] In fact, the Minnesota state epidemiologist, Michael Osterholm, concluded that the Hib vaccine *increases* the risk of illness.[134] But the Minnesota data was conveniently excluded by at least one Hib researcher who had the responsibility of submitting impartial conclusions to vaccine policymakers.[135]

Doctors have been warned by the CDC that cases of Hib may occur after vaccination, "prior to the onset of the protective effects of the vaccine."[136] Other studies warn of "increased susceptibility" to the disease during the first seven days after vaccination.[137] The AAP notes that the vaccine is not expected to protect the child for up to three weeks after receiving the shot. They tell doctors to warn parents to look for signs of the disease in their children following vaccination.[138] In one study of 55 children who contracted Hib at least three weeks after vaccination, 39 developed meningitis.[139]

According to Dr. Stephen L. Coeni, an official at the CDC, nearly 70 percent of all Hib cases in children 18 months and older are contracted at day care centers.[140] So when the Hib vaccine was licensed for use in the United States, the disease it was meant to protect against was hyped as being extremely contagious. However, in two separate studies, researchers found that the disease does not spread easily. Out of 772 children who came into contact with an infected child, none of the 185 children in the first study, and only one of the 587 children in the second study, caught the disease.[141]

Because of the controversy over the safety and efficacy of the vaccine, the AAP approved new guidelines recommending that doctors use their own discretion regarding whether or not to continue giving the Hib vaccine to children.[142]

"Conjugated" Hib: In 1988 a new "conjugated" Hib vaccine was approved for use in children at least 18 months old. By 1991 its recommended use was extended to infants as young as two months. Today it is mandated in at least 44 states.[143]

The conjugated vaccine is expensive and its protection is temporary. Thus, doctors are recommending four shots: three doses two months apart, beginning at two months, and another booster shot at 15 months.[144]

Officials are concerned about an increased chance of acquiring Hib during the first several days after receiving the shot.[145]

Hepatitis B: Hepatitis is a liver disease usually accompanied by a fever and caused by a virus. High-risk groups include sexually active homosexual men, prostitutes, and IV drug users. Infants and children rarely develop this disease.[146] Still, in 1991 the CDC and AAP began the process of mandating this vaccine for all infants. Today, many babies receive multiple doses beginning at birth.

A study by the Institute of Medicine found that recipients of the plasma-derived hepatitis B vaccine may have received shots contaminated with HIV, a precursor to AIDS.[147] Two thirds of doctors eligible for the hepatitis vaccine refused to take it, and 87 percent do not believe it is needed by their newborn patients.[148,149]

In France, hundreds of people suffered from autoimmune and neurological disorders, including multiple sclerosis, following hepatitis B vaccines. As a result, in October 1998 France ended the mandatory hepatitis B vaccine program for all school children.[150]

Numerous studies throughout the world question the safety and efficacy of the hepatitis B vaccine.[151]

Influenza (Swine Flu, Russian Flu, Asian Flu, etc.): The safety and efficacy of the flu vaccine is debatable, especially since the strains covered by one year's vaccine rarely correspond to the strains causing the flu at the present time.[152]

In 1976 more than 500 people who received their flu shots were paralyzed with Guillain-Barre syndrome. Thirty of them died. During that same year, the incidence of Guillain-Barre among flu-vaccinated U.S. Army personnel was 50 percent greater than among unvaccinated civilians. Dr. John Seal of the National Institute of Allergy and Infectious Disease believes that "any and all flu vaccines are capable of causing Guillain-Barre."[153]

In a recent study, half of all elderly people who requested a flu vaccine were discouraged against it by their doctors.[154]

Pneumonia: The *Journal of Infectious Diseases* published a controlled study on the pneumonia vaccine using 1300 healthy children. Some of the children received the vaccine; others were given a placebo. Conclusion: there is no benefit. Recipients of the vaccine had "no fewer days of respiratory illness, no reduction in antibiotic consumption, hospitalization, visits to a physician, or incidence of ear infections" when compared to the control group.[155]

Chickenpox: A chickenpox vaccine has been available for years, but authorities have been reluctant to promote it. For one thing, the vaccine is a weakened form of the virus, which may be harbored in the body indefinitely. For another, long-term studies have not been conducted. In addition, naturally occurring chickenpox tends to confer lifelong immunity; thus, any failure of the vaccine to offer sustained protection could increase the recipients' vulnerability to the disease during adulthood, when complications are more likely and more serious.[156]

A 1985 CDC study determined that the medical costs involved in treating chickenpox did not warrant the expenditures required to promote a national vaccine program. Nevertheless, in 1995 it was licensed for use in the United States, and is now being added to mandatory vaccine schedules in several states, because "the U.S. could save five times as much as it would spend on the vaccine" by avoiding the costs incurred by moms and dads who stay home to care for their sick children.[157]

Smallpox: Official statistics from many countries indicate that smallpox (and other communicable diseases) were declining before vaccination programs were enforced. This may be attributed to the sanitation reforms and nutritional teachings instituted around the mid-1800's. For example, water supplies were protected from contamination, streets and stables were cleaned, sewage was removed, and food was delivered while still fresh. However, once smallpox vaccinations became mandatory, deaths from the disease steadily increased. In fact, records in several countries show that nearly every contagious disease — plague, cholera, measles, scarlet fever, dysentery, whooping cough — *except smallpox* (kept alive by mandatory shots), declined in number and severity on its own.[158]

Before England passed a compulsory vaccination law in 1853, the highest death rate for any two year period was only 2,000 cases, even during the most severe epidemics.[159] (Jenner himself admitted that smallpox was relatively unknown before he began his vaccinations.[160] In fact, there were only a few hundred cases of smallpox in England at that time)[161] After more than fifteen years of mandatory vaccinations, in 1870 and 1871 alone more than 23,000 people died from the disease.[162] In Germany, over 124,000 people died of smallpox during the same epidemic. All had been vaccinated.[163] In Japan, nearly 29,000 people died in just seven years under a stringent compulsory vaccination and re-vaccination program.[164] Compare these devastating figures to Australia, where the government terminated compulsory vaccinations when two children died from their smallpox shots. As a result, smallpox virtually disappeared in that country (three cases in fifteen years).[165]

Figure 11:

SMALLPOX DEATHS TUMBLED ONLY
AFTER PEOPLE REFUSED THE SHOTS
(Figures represent official statistics from England and Wales)

Ten Year Period Ending:	% of Babies Vaccinated:	Smallpox Deaths (per million):
1881	96.5	3708
1891	82.1	933
1901	67.9	437
1911	67.6	395
1921	42.3	12
1931	43.1	25
1941	39.9	1

Every examination of the facts indicates that the smallpox vaccine was not only ineffective but dangerous. Undoctored hospital records consistently show that about 90 percent of all smallpox cases occurred after the individual was vaccinated.[166] "Deaths certified as due to vaccination...have several times outnumbered those from smallpox." — Dr. Millard, Medical Officer of Health.[167] But hospital records often were doctored, and death certificates were falsified when patients died of smallpox after vaccination.[168] "The credit of vaccination is kept up statistically by diagnosing all the [cases of smallpox after vaccinations] as pustular eczema [or anything else] except smallpox." — London Health Official.[169]

There is a direct relationship between the percentage of babies vaccinated and the number of smallpox deaths: the higher the percentage, the greater the fatalities. In other words, deaths from smallpox tumbled only after people refused the shots (Figure 11).[170]

Multiple vaccinations against smallpox were common. However, a study published in 1980 by *Mutation Research* showed that children who were re-vaccinated against smallpox had "chromosomal aberrations in their white blood cells." The authors of this study concluded that smallpox vaccination has a "mutagenic effect" on human chromosomes.[171] (For more information on vaccines and Genetic Mutation, see page 48 on this topic.)

Note: James Phipps, the eight-year-old boy initially vaccinated by Jenner in 1796, was re-vaccinated 20 times, and died at the age of twenty. Jenner's own son, who was also vaccinated more than once, died at twenty-one. Both succumbed to tuberculosis, a condition that some researchers have linked to the smallpox vaccine.[172]

LONG-TERM EFFECTS

Few serious attempts have been made to discover the long-term effects of injecting foreign proteins and toxic substances into the healthy bodies of innocent infants. In fact, research focusing on possible correlations between vaccines and autoimmune diseases, and neurologically-based disorders (i.e., multiple sclerosis, cerebral palsy, Guillain-Barre syndrome, cancer, AIDS) is just beginning. For example, one medical researcher, Dr. Richard Moskowitz, recently concluded that the unnatural process of vaccination can lead to slow viruses developing in the body. These may bring about the "far less curable chronic diseases of the present."[173] He also noted that "these illnesses may be considerably more serious than the original disease, involving deeper structures [and] more vital organs."[174] Other researchers have identified an actual "lowering of the body's resistance resulting from vaccinations." They warn us about the "probability of widespread and unrecognized vaccine-induced immune system malfunction." They also note that this effect is often delayed, indirect, and masked, its true nature seldom recognized.[175]

The Immune System: Several researchers have noted that vaccines merely "trick" the body into focusing on only one aspect (antibody production) of the many complex and integrated strategies normally available to the immune system. Diseases contracted naturally are ordinarily filtered through a series of immune system defenses. But when the vaccine virus is injected directly into the child's blood stream, it gains access to all of the major tissues and organs of the body *without the body's normal advantage of a total immune response.*[176] Antibodies (T-lymphocytes) that do respond to the invading vaccine germs become committed to those germs and are unable to react to other challenges to the health of the child.[177,178]

Research indicates that the immature immune system of a baby is stimulated, strengthened, and matured by responding to *natural* challenges. When the infant gains exposure to viral and bacterial microorganisms *in the environment*, normal development of the immune system is likely to occur. However, if the immature immune system is forced to respond to a barrage of vaccinations injected directly into the body, bypassing outer immune system defenses, inner immune system protective maneuvers may be overwhelmed. When natural immunity is curtailed and the immune system compelled to operate in unnatural ways, questions arise regarding its ability to protect the child throughout life.[179]

The immune system is designed to help the organism discriminate "self" from everything else that is foreign and potentially dangerous to the "self." Under natural conditions, enemy germs are attacked and rendered benign by the immune system. But alien viruses injected into the body fuse with healthy cells, and continue to replicate along with those cells.[180] This is likely to confuse the immune system, which can no longer differentiate between harmful and harmless conditions within the body. Under these circumstances, the immune system is likely to either invade its own cells (cancer), or ignore danger signs altogether, leaving the organism vulnerable to any number of autoimmune diseases.[181]

Autopsies were performed comparing the thymus glands (responsible for the production of protective T-cells) of adults in poorly vaccinated countries versus adults in the United States. They found that in the U.S. thymus glands begin to atrophy following puberty; thymus gland deterioration was found to be minimal in adults from the poorly vaccinated countries. Thymus gland abnormalities are associated with a variety of autoimmune and tumor producing diseases (e.g., many different types of cancer, leukemia, lupus erythematosus, and rheumatoid arthritis). Some researchers blame this situation on the widespread, mandatory childhood vaccination programs.[182]

Genetic Mutation: The polio vaccine contains monkey kidney cell culture and calf serum. The MMR (measles, mumps, and rubella) vaccine is prepared in chick embryo. Monkey kidney, calf serum, and chick embryo are foreign proteins — biological matter composed of animal cells. Because they are injected directly into the bloodstream, they are able to change our genetic structure.[183,184]

Viruses (and viral vaccines) are agents for the transfer of genetic imprints from one host to another. In other words, because they contain pure genetic material (DNA and RNA) from a foreign organism, once injected into a human recipient, the new genetic material is incorporated into the invaded cells.[185]

There is a lot of literature confirming the action of viruses in bringing about genetic changes in unrelated organisms.[186,187] As early as the 1950's Barbara McClintock, an American genetic scientist, described the behavior of mobile genetic elements — "jumping genes."[188] And in the 1960's Joshua Lederberg, from the Department of Genetics, Stanford University School of Medicine, notified the scientific world that "live viruses are...genetic messages used for the purpose of programming human cells." He was also notably explicit when he said that "we already practice biological engineering on a rather large scale by use of live viruses in mass immunization campaigns."[189]

No one knows the long-term effects of tampering with the genetic codes and delicate structure of the human organism. However, the physical invasion of the human body by foreign genetic material may have the immediate effect of permanently weakening the immune system, setting in motion a new era of autoimmune diseases.[190] For example, research indicates that psychotic disorders may be caused by viral infections.[191-193] The incidence of schizophrenia is on the rise compared to earlier times,[194] and studies now indicate that about one-third of all cases are autoimmune in nature.[195] Once again, some authorities implicate the childhood vaccine programs.[196]

AIDS: During the 1950's and 1960's millions of people were injected with polio vaccines that were contaminated with the SV-40 virus (undetected in the Simian monkey organs used to prepare the vaccines).[197-204] SV-40 is considered a powerful immunosuppressor and trigger for HIV — the name given to the AIDS virus. It is said to cause a clinical condition indistinguishable from AIDS, and has been found in brain tumors, leukemia, and other human cancers as well. Researchers consider it to be a cancer-causing virus.[205]

Esteemed polio researcher, Dr. Hilary Koprowski, has warned congressmen that "an almost infinite number of monkey viruses" can contaminate polio vaccines.[206] In fact, the genetic sequences of some monkey viruses are as close to some strains of the AIDS virus as some strains of the AIDS virus are to each other.[207] But tests to determine the existence of some of these viruses were not developed until the mid-1980's. This makes it extremely likely that these viruses contaminated vaccines in the 1960's and 1970's, before virus detection techniques were refined.[208] And at least one health official has voiced the obvious regarding our knowledge of animal viruses and the status of vaccines today: "You can't test for something if you don't know it's there."[209]

In a recent article published in the British medical journal *Lancet*, the author noted that the oral polio vaccine — which was also used experimentally during the mid-1970's to treat recurrent herpes — was probably contaminated with a number of potentially dangerous retroviruses. The use of this vaccine for experimental purposes may have seeded HIV among American homosexuals.[210]

Scientists and other researchers have uncovered a link between the smallpox vaccine and AIDS. According to Dr. Robert Gallo, the chief AIDS researcher at the National Cancer Institute, "the use of live vaccines such as that used for smallpox can activate a dormant infection such as HIV." In fact, the greatest spread of HIV infection coincides with the most intense and recent smallpox vaccination campaigns. Information on the seven Central African countries most infected with AIDS — Zaire, Zambia, Tanzania, Uganda, Malawai, Ruandi, and Burundi — precisely matches WHO figures indicating the number of people vaccinated. Brazil, the only South American country included in the smallpox campaign, has the greatest incidence of AIDS on that continent.[211]

In Central Africa (where the AIDS epidemic is thought to have originated) AIDS was more evenly spread among males and females than in the West. But about 14,000 Haitians were in Central Africa on a United Nations assignment when the smallpox campaign took place. They were also vaccinated against smallpox, and began to return home at a time when Haiti had become a popular getaway for San Francisco homosexuals.[212]

In 1969, the U.S. Department of Defense sought funds from Congress to create a "synthetic biological agent, an agent that does not naturally exist and for which no natural immunity could have been acquired."[213] In a controversial article published by *Health Freedom News*, William Campbell Douglass, MD, claims that this virus — the AIDS virus — was deliberately manufactured by the National Cancer Institute in collaboration with the World Health Organization.[214] He supports this assertion with direct quotes from a bulletin published by WHO in 1972. Evidently, they wanted to create a hybrid virus in an attempt "to ascertain whether viruses can in fact exert selective effects on immune function."[215] He describes research into how these organizations combined two deadly retroviruses — bovine leukemia virus (BLV) and sheep visna virus — to create the AIDS virus. (Some retroviruses may take up to 40 years to manifest.)[216] Dr. Douglass asserts that during official proceedings in 1972, WHO suggested that a useful way to study the effects of the new virus would be to put it into a vaccination program and observe the results. He and other researchers claim WHO used the smallpox vaccine for this study and chose Central Africa to begin.[217]

Needles were reused 40 to 60 times during the Central African smallpox vaccine campaign. The primary method of sterilization consisted of waving the needle across a flame. Needle-sharing contributes to the transmission of infectious disease.[218]

Note: Immoral, unethical, and illegal medical experimentation still occurs. For example, in December of 1990 a federal regulation was adopted permitting the Food and Drug Administration (FDA) to circumvent U.S. and international laws forbidding medical experiments on unwilling subjects. This regulation permits the FDA to inject American troops with unapproved experimental drugs or vaccines *without their informed consent.* The FDA merely needs to deem it "not feasible" to obtain the soldier's permission.[219]

Dr. William Douglass also acknowledges that AIDS was brought into the United States from Haiti by homosexuals, but implicates the hepatitis B vaccine for the sudden proliferation of AIDS in the homosexual population. (The hepatitis B vaccine exhibits the exact epidemiology as AIDS.) He notes that a Dr. W. Schmugner, head of the New York City blood bank, set up the rules for the hepatitis vaccine studies. Only males between the ages of 20 and 40, *who were not monogamous*, were allowed to participate. Because all vaccine recipients in the study were required to be promiscuous, Dr. Douglass speculates that there was a deliberate attempt to spread something among the population. Although this information appears fantastic, in 1981 the CDC reported that four percent of those receiving the hepatitis vaccine were AIDS infected. In 1984 the CDC acknowledged that the true figure is 60 percent. By 1987 they refused to give out any figures at all.[220]

Finally, even though several plausible theories linking vaccines to AIDS have been offered, health officials remain obstinately opposed, even hostile, to suggestions that further investigations be made. Dr. David Heymann, head of the Office of Research for the World Health Organization's Global Program on AIDS, stubbornly insisted that "any speculation on how [the AIDS virus] arose is of no importance."[221] And even though the original seed stocks of the polio vaccines from the early 1960's are available, the FDA claims they were never tested, even by WHO. According to the FDA, this is because there are not enough vials of the material, and testing "might use it all up."[222]

Developmental Disabilities: According to the medical historian, Harris L. Coulter, Ph.D., "the family and society are both victims of vaccination programs forced on them by state legislatures that are entirely too responsive to medical opinion and medical organizations." The entire postwar American generation is suffering from what he calls "post-encephalitic syndrome" (PES) — the name he gives to define a variety of vaccine-induced disabilities.[223] To support his assertions, Coulter presented evidence showing that the long-term effects of vaccinations may be more pervasive than suspected. However, disabilities caused by the vaccines are often "disguised" under different names: autism, dyslexia, learning disability, epilepsy, mental retardation, hyperactivity, and minimal brain dysfunction, to name a few. Juvenile delinquency, an unprecedented rise in violent crime, drug abuse, and the collapse of the American school system unable to contend with the estimated 20 to 25 percent of students mentally and emotionally deficient, represent other conditions that may be attributed to the vaccines.[224]

Post-Vaccinal Encephalitis: The developmental disabilities and other conditions noted above are frequently caused by encephalitis, or inflammation of the brain. Medical practitioners know that encephalitis can be caused by a severe injury to the head, a severe burn, from an infectious disease, *or from the vaccines against these diseases* — post-vaccinal encephalitis.[225] *The principal cause of encephalitis in the United States today, and in other industrialized countries, is the childhood vaccination program.*[226]

The symptoms of post-vaccinal encephalitis are identical to the symptoms of encephalitis arising from any other cause.[227] Since any segment of the nervous system may be affected, every possible physical, intellectual, and personality deviation, and combinations of them, are possible.[228,229]

Autopsies after post-vaccinal encephalitis show a loss and destruction of myelin on the brainstem and spinal cord. Myelin covers and protects the nerves much like the insulation on an electric wire. Without myelin, nerve impulses are short-circuited and the nervous system remains undeveloped and immature.[230]

An overt reaction to the vaccine is not required to confirm that damage to the central nervous system was caused by post-vaccinal encephalitis. In fact, there is no correlation between the degree of cerebral damage that may later ensue and the severity of the condition that lead to encephalitis in the first place.[231-236] In other words, subtle and often overlooked reactions to the vaccine (i.e., a slight fever, fussiness, drowsiness) can be, and often is, a case of encephalitis which is capable of causing severe neurological complications months or even years later.[237]

Now let's look at some of the specific disabilities that may be attributed to post-vaccinal encephalitis:

Autism: In 1943 the well known child psychiatrist, Leo Kanner, announced his discovery of eleven cases of a new mental disorder. He noted that "the condition differs markedly and uniquely from anything reported so far..."[238] This condition soon became known as autism. (Autism is a form of childhood schizophrenia.

Children with this disorder are frequently retarded, mute, and unresponsive to human contact.) These first cases of autism in the United States occurred at a time when the pertussis vaccine was becoming increasingly available. By the 1950's and 1960's parents from all over the country were seeking help for their autistic children. The growing numbers of children suffering from this new illness directly coincided with the growing popularity of the mandated vaccination programs during these same years. Today, over 4500 new cases of autism occur every year in the U.S. alone.[239]

The same correlations between autism and childhood vaccination programs may be found in other countries as well. In Japan, the first autistic child was diagnosed in 1945.[240] When the United States ended the war and occupied Japan, a mandatory vaccination program was established. Today, hundreds of new cases of autism are diagnosed in Japanese children every year.[241]

Europe received the pertussis vaccine in the 1950's; the first cases of autism began to appear there in the same decade. In England the pertussis vaccine wasn't promoted on a large scale until the late 1950's. Shortly thereafter, in 1962, the National Society for Autistic Children in Britain was established.[242]

When the first cases of autism began to appear, researchers were puzzled by the high incidence of autistic children being born into well-educated families. Over 90 percent of the parents were high-school graduates. Nearly three-fourths of the fathers and one-half of the mothers had graduated from college. Many had professional careers. As a result, scientists unsuccessfully tried to link autism to genetic factors in the upper-class populations.[243] Meanwhile, psychiatrists, unaware of the neurological basis of the illness, sought psychological explanations. The mother, especially, was blamed for her restrained emotions.[244,245]

Today in the United States autism is evenly distributed among all social classes and ethnic groups. Socioeconomic disparities began to disappear during the 1970's.[246] Once again this puzzled the researchers. Many simply concluded that earlier studies were flawed. But there is an explanation.

When the pertussis vaccine was initially introduced, only the rich and educated parents who sought the very best for their children, and who could afford a private doctor, were in a position to request the newest medical advancements. Free vaccinations at public health clinics didn't yet exist. And compulsory vaccination programs were still on the horizon. But as vaccine programs grew, parents from across the socioeconomic spectrum gained equal access to them. Thus, autistic children were now being discovered within every kind of family, and in dreadfully greater numbers than ever before imagined.[247]

Hyperactivity/Minimal Brain Dysfunction: In the 1950's another disorder rapidly spread among school children and gained prominence in the medical science and health literature: hyperactivity (attention-deficit hyperactivity disorder — ADHD). In 1963 the U.S. Public Health Service listed dozens of symptoms associated with hyperactivity and officially changed the name to "minimal brain dysfunction" (MBD). By the 1970's some leading authorities noted that this disorder appeared to lie at the root of nearly every type of childhood behavior problem, and had become the most commonly diagnosed illness among child guidance counselors.[248] In 1988 the *Journal of the American Medical Association* acknowledged that minimal brain damage had become the leading disability reported by elementary schools, and "one of the most common referral problems to child psychiatry outpatient clinics."[249]

In some school districts as many as thirteen percent of the children are now enrolled in "special education classes."[250] But minimally brain damaged children often go undetected, and some researchers have indicated that the actual figures for children with this disorder are closer to fifteen to twenty percent.[251]

Although many children are not diagnosed as learning disabled or minimally brain damaged, teachers complain that nearly all of their students are cognitively inferior and have shorter attention spans when compared to kids they taught in the 1960's.[252] One instructor notes that when she gives directions many forget them almost immediately, even after several repetitions. "They look around, fidget, and doodle." Another teacher laments that "kids' brains must be different these days."[253] In fact, beginning in 1964 the average SAT verbal and math scores have continued to steadily decline.[254] In an attempt to appease school administrators, who are often blamed for declining scores, and to safeguard the truth, test-makers have been "dumbing down" their tests since the 1960's. Our children today are taking tests drastically more simple than those given decades ago.[255]

Like autism, minimal brain dysfunction was initially thought to have psychological origins. But these children usually exhibit symptoms associated with neurological damage: seizure disorders, tics, tremors, infantile spasms, EEG abnormalities, motor impairments, poor visual-motor coordination, and cranial nerve palsies (capable of causing visual defects, eye disturbances, and hearing and speech impediments).[256]

A few brief examples of the neurological basis for minimal brain dysfunction are given below:

MBD Case #1: Harold reacted to his 2nd DPT shot with a 104 degree fever and high-pitched screaming (recall the similarity to the cri encephalique, or the encephalitic scream associated with central nervous system damage). Harold is now blind.[257]

MBD Case #2: Kate was four months old when she received the DPT shot. Within 72 hours she was shrieking in pain. Today she continues to have seizures and cannot speak.[258]

MBD Case #3: Judy had her first grand mal seizure seven days after her 2nd DPT shot. Today she has a very low attention span and tends to reverse letters and write things backwards.[259]

MBD Case #4: Ralph reacted to his first three DPT shots with persistent crying and a 104 degree fever. Today he has visual perception problems and cannot read or write correctly.[260]

MBD Case #5: Wayne reacted to his fifth DPT shot with screams, a 104 degree fever, by rocking from side to side, and hallucinating. Today he is dyslexic.[261]

MBD Case #6: On the fourth day after 6-year-old Cassidy received her measles shot, she turned deathly ill and collapsed following a seizure. Today she is developmentally delayed.[262]

MBD Case #7: Within hours after Daniel received his 2nd DPT shot he began screaming, turned rigid, and went limp. Since then, he has suffered from daily seizures. Today he is physically and developmentally disabled.[263]

MBD Case #8: Wesley reacted to his 2nd DPT shot with glazed eyes and seizures. Today he continues to have up to 30 seizures daily, and has been diagnosed as permanently brain damaged.[264]

Violent Crime: A disproportionate amount of violent crime is committed by individuals with neurological damage.[265] For example, as early as the 1920's researchers were aware that children who had "recovered" from encephalitis were more likely to appear troubled and engage in abusive, cruel, and destructive behavior. Such children were often called "apaches."[266,267] Today we call these children juvenile delinquents (suffering from hyperactivity and conduct disorder), but their numbers are now of epidemic proportions and their crimes are more violent.[268]

Dyslexia and other learning disabilities have been found in nearly 90 percent of delinquents.[269] Delinquent children with these disorders often become sociopaths upon reaching adulthood.[270]

Studies confirm that children with neurological disorders often engage in violent criminal behavior as adolescents and adults. In one study of hyperactive children it was discovered that they were 20 times more likely than the rest of the population to end up in a reform school.[271] In another study, half of the imprisoned delinquents had an IQ below 85.[272] In 1988 the *Journal of the American Medical Association* acknowledged that a disproportionate number of felons suffered from hyperactivity during their earlier years.[273]

Epilepsy and seizure disorders frequently occur following cases of post-vaccinal encephalitis. Studies indicate that epileptics find it significantly more difficult to control their impulses and aggressiveness.[274] In one study, the number of prisoners with a history of seizures was found to be nearly ten times greater than the general population.[275] In another study of 321 middle class, extremely violent individuals, more than 90 percent showed evidence of brain damage, including a medical history implicating epilepsy.[276]

Drug Abuse: Psychiatrists and pediatricians prescribe a variety of drugs to young children in their attempts to control the effects of hyperactivity and minimal brain dysfunction. In one study it was estimated that 6 percent of American schoolchildren rely on these compounds to render them "manageable." But in some communities where doctors "specialize" in these disorders, the percentage is much greater.[277] Many of these drugs — from tranquilizers to antipsychotics — have adverse side-effects that are considered by some researchers to be worse than the original symptoms. These new symptoms are sometimes irreversible.[278]

Many parents and other individuals who have studied the above problems believe that the medical abuse of drugs in school children predisposes them to abuse "street drugs" later in life.[279]

Adolescents suffering from minimal brain dysfunction are high risk for engaging in unusually early smoking, drinking, and substance abuse.[280] Adults with this disorder are also notably susceptible to alcoholism and the misuse of drugs.[281]

Note: The very latest studies linking vaccines to new diseases, including autism, diabetes and multiple sclerosis, may be found in my new book, *Vaccine Reactions: The Hidden Epidemic.* I also recommend visiting the *Thinktwice Global Vaccine Institute* website for additional information: www.thinktwice.com

MORE VACCINE INFORMATION

The National Childhood Vaccine Injury Act of 1986, Public Law 99-660, is a federal law passed by Congress that was created to officially recognize the reality of vaccine-caused injuries and death. The law contains two main elements: safety provisions, and a no-fault federal compensation program.

The safety reform portion of the law...
1. requires doctors to provide parents with information about childhood diseases and vaccines prior to vaccination. (See the section on Vaccine Contraindications.)
2. requires all doctors who administer vaccines to report vaccine reactions to federal health officials. (See the section on Reporting Vaccine Reactions.)
3. requires doctors to record vaccine reactions in an individual's permanent record.
4. requires doctors to keep a record of the date that each vaccine was given, the manufacturer's name and lot number, where the vaccine was administered, and the professional title (M.D., R.N.) of the person administering the vaccine.
5. mandates that the federal government promote the improvement of existing vaccines and develop safer vaccines. (See the section on Promoting Vaccine Safety.)

The compensation portion of the law...
1. is an alternative to suing vaccine manufacturers and physicians when children or adults are damaged or die from reactions to mandated vaccines.
2. awards up to $250,000 if the individual dies, or for pain and suffering in the case of a living (but brain damaged) child.[282] (See the section on Claims For Compensation.)

Vaccine Contraindications — High Risk Individuals: Very few doctors inform parents about vaccine risks. But vaccine manufacturers place warnings in vaccine containers indicating who *should not* receive vaccinations. The American Academy of Pediatrics (AAP), and the Department of Health and Human Services (HHS) also make recommendations indicating who *should not* receive vaccinations. (The AAP publishes a _Report of the Committee on Infectious Diseases_ every four years; HHS has guidelines formulated by the Advisory Committee on Immunization Practices (ACIP), which appear in the _Morbidity and Mortality Report_ published by the CDC). This information is included below:

POLIO: Children younger than 6 weeks; people who are ill, or who have cancer of the lymph system.

MEASLES: Children younger than 15 months; pregnant women; people who are ill, or who are allergic to eggs, chicken, feathers, or who have cancer, blood disease, or deficiencies of the immune system.

RUBELLA: Pregnant women; people who are allergic to eggs, chicken, duck, or feathers, or who have cancer, blood disease, or deficiencies of the immune system.

DPT: Any child past the 7th birthday, or who has had a severe reaction to a previous dose, or who has a personal history of convulsions or neurological disease, or who is acutely sick with a fever or respiratory infection, or who is taking medication that may suppress the immune system.[283]

The three vaccine policymakers in America, noted above, do not "officially" consider the following conditions contraindications to the DPT vaccine. However, scientific literature published by pertussis vaccine researchers throughout the world for the past 40 years indicates that such conditions may put a child at high risk:

1. The child is ill with anything, including a runny nose, cough, ear infection, diarrhea, or has recovered from an illness within one month prior to a scheduled DPT shot.
2. The child has a family member who had a severe reaction to a DPT shot.
3. Someone in the child's immediate family has a history of convulsions or neurological disease.
4. The child was born prematurely or with low birthweight.
5. The child has a personal or family history of severe allergies (i.e., cow's milk, asthma, eczema).[284]

Vaccines may also be contraindicated for certain people with special conditions not listed above. If you suspect that you or your child may be at high risk, **_Get The Facts!_**

Reporting Vaccine Reactions: Many doctors refuse to report vaccine reactions to health authorities despite the legal requirement to do so. According to Barbara Loe Fisher, executive vice president of the National Vaccine Information Center (NVIC), "the will and intent of Congress in enacting the National Vaccine Injury Act of 1986 is being subverted. This subversion is resulting in an appalling underreporting of vaccine reactions and deaths by both private and public health physicians... [There is also] a lack of recordkeeping and/or willingness on the part of physicians to divulge the manufacturer's name and lot number when a reaction occurs."[285]

According to NVIC, doctors often justify their refusal to report vaccine reactions by merely claiming the shot had nothing to do with the child's injury or death. Some pediatricians may actually believe this, because they quote vaccine policymakers in the AAP and CDC who tell them that the vaccine is completely safe.[286] However, the fear of being sued for failing to warn parents of the potential dangers and contraindications may also be a consideration.

The following excerpts from parents and relatives of vaccine-damaged children illustrate how doctors can easily dismiss apparent vaccine reactions and thus justify not reporting them:

Excerpt: "Our son had his 2nd DPT shot and oral polio [vaccine] at four months of age on September 22, 1989. He had reacted to his 1st DPT immunization two months earlier with prolonged high-pitched screaming and projectile vomiting... After his 2nd shot he immediately started the high-pitched screaming again. He could no longer hold his head up and could not keep his food down. He couldn't sleep or stay awake, he had absence seizures, dozens to hundreds a day. He deteriorated daily and died April 14, 1990." *The doctor would not report this reaction. He did not feel that it was related to the vaccine.*

Excerpt: "Our 16 month old grandson received his 4th DPT shot on December 5, 1989, and he died 24 days later. He also received the MMR and oral polio vaccine at the same time. Within 24 hours his legs were red and swollen, he had a fever of 103 degrees, and he was very fussy and irritable... His previous shots had similar reactions... We know the shot contributed to his death." *The doctor would not report this reaction. He did not feel that it was related to the vaccine.*

Excerpt: "We lost our beautiful, precious and adored four month old son 26 hours after receiving the DPT vaccination and oral polio [vaccine] at his well-baby check-up on January 25, 1990... We were aware our son's behavior patterns changed after the shot... He was staring, looked spacey, only took short naps, vomited his bottle... The doctor was insistent that this was a SIDS death." *The doctor would not report this reaction. He did not feel that it was related to the vaccine.*

Excerpt: "Our son had his 1st DPT vaccination and oral polio vaccine at 14 months old on February 22, 1990. That evening he started high-pitched screaming. The next two days he had a temperature of 101 degrees and slept for 15 hours. When he awoke he was extremely irritable... My son was in a lot of body pain. At times he looked like he had a stroke. At other times he was curled up in a hard knot we couldn't straighten. He was having seizures and we didn't know it... He continues to have seizures. The doctor, even though law required him to record manufacturer and lot number, did not record the number..." *The doctor would not report this reaction. He did not feel that it was related to the vaccine.*

Excerpt: "My son had his first DPT shot at his two month check-up on May 8, 1990... Four hours later he started crying... I noticed he was pale and like a statue... He stopped breathing. I picked him up and shook him and he started breathing again. A friend was visiting and called 911. He stopped breathing 8-10 more times with me shaking him out of it each time before the paramedics arrived. He was ash white...screaming when we got to the hospital... I have another child who had severe reactions from his shots. He had a seizure after each of his first three DPT shots and was on medication for three years." *The doctor would not report this reaction. He did not feel that it was related to the vaccine.*

Excerpt: "My sixteen month old grandson had his 2nd DPT shot, MMR and Polio at his well-baby check-up on August 16, 1990. In less than 48 hours he had a temperature of 105 degrees and went into convulsions... My grandson has deteriorated daily. He walks stiff-legged or his knee collapses on under him... He has trouble with his bowels, constipation one minute followed by diarrhea running down his leg the next minute. We look at our old videos and realize how much he has changed." *The doctor would not report this reaction, nor would he give the parents the manufacturers and lot numbers of the vaccines he administered.*

Excerpt: "My grandson had his 1st DPT shot and oral polio [vaccine] at his two month well-baby check-up on June 8, 1990. Within 21 hours he was dead. After the shot he started crying [high-pitched screaming]... My grandson began projectile vomiting and continued the high-pitched crying... At 7 A.M. my daughter awoke and found my grandson to have a purple color on one side of his face, clenched fists, blood coming from his nose and mouth and not breathing. My grandson was dead. I have promised my daughter that his death will not be in vain and just another statistic labeled

SIDS." *The doctor would not report this reaction. He did not feel that it was related to the vaccine.*[287]

Note: If the doctor or pediatrician does not report the vaccine reaction, parents should file their own report: 1-800-822-7967.

What Causes a Vaccine Reaction? When children receive their shots from a "hot lot" (an improperly prepared and dangerous batch of vaccine that bypassed the safety testing system) they are especially susceptible to the inherent risks of the vaccine. For example, in 1975 the state of Michigan sent a batch of the DPT vaccine to the FDA for testing. The FDA found the entire lot to be three times more potent than regulations allowed. Instead of immediately destroying the bad lot, Michigan health authorities decided to "test" it on hundreds of children in their state. This had disastrous results. (Later, when the parents of children who were paralyzed and brain damaged from the "hot lot" tried to sue the state, the courts disallowed their case because the "doctrine of sovereign immunity" protects the government from claims arising from services that only the government can provide.)[288]

Several studies indicate that children do not have to receive a shot from a "hot lot" in order to be at risk. Instead, certain children appear to be "anatomically susceptible," or genetically predisposed to having a reaction to the vaccine.[289,290]

Many parents are unaware that potentially dangerous reactions even exist, so they fail to remain alert for neurological signs and other symptoms in their babies following their shots. However, in one study, when parents were asked to specifically observe any change in their baby's behavior or physical condition after a shot, only seven percent reported no reactions at all.[291]

Where Do Coroners Stand? Doctors and pediatricians are not the only instruments of the Medical-Industrial Complex who have been known to deny the existence of vaccine reactions and cover up the truth. The medically trained coroners are also members of this elite group. Many are highly skilled in the art of subterfuge. Rarely is the vaccination ever listed as the cause of death. Instead, they use impressive terms to falsify death certificates: cardiac arrest, possible myocarditis; bronchial bilateral pneumonia;[292] septicemia due to septic tonsillitis; lymphatic leukemia; streptococcal cellulitis; tubercular meningitis; infantile paralysis; and SIDS, to name a few.[293]

When one mother, whose son died four days after his second polio shot, studied his "provisional" autopsy report, she noted that there were major findings of myocarditis, and hepatitis, and that the polio virus had been isolated in his diseased organs — conditions not inconsistent with a vaccine reaction. But when she questioned the pathology department's initial conclusion — Sudden Infant Death Syndrome — and requested additional tests to determine whether the polio virus was a wild or vaccine strain, she was led into a nine year battle with the CDC to secure the results.

Note: Medical authorities were forced to concede the truth. The official death certificate listed the cause of death as "myocarditis, due to type 2 polio virus, due to oral Sabin polio vaccine."[294]

Promoting Vaccine Safety: The National Vaccine Advisory Committee (NVAC) was created by the Department of Health and Human Services (HHS), after Congress ordered HHS "to develop and disseminate vaccine information materials for distribution by health care providers." This material was to include information on adverse reactions, contraindications, and the availability of a federal no-fault compensation program for those who are injured or die from a mandated vaccine. Congress believed then, as it does now, that parents are entitled to such information before their children receive vaccinations.

HHS was to satisfy this legal requirement by no later than December 22, 1988. However, by March 4, 1991, this matter was still unsettled, and notice was provided to Louis W. Sullivan, M.D., secretary of HHS, of the intent to bring a lawsuit against Sullivan and the Department for failure to perform an "act or duty" as required by law. This notice was submitted by NVIC on behalf of several parents of vaccination-aged children.[295]

Because HHS has failed to publish the required information, high risk children who *should not* receive one or more of the vaccines may suffer from avoidable brain damage, permanent disabilities, and even death. And parents whose children were injured or died from one or more of the vaccines during the past few years may still be unaware of their right to seek compensation.

Vaccine guidelines were eventually submitted by the advisory committee (after the December 22, 1988 deadline) but were rejected by NVIC on the grounds that they "failed to meet even minimal standards of scientific rigor, candor, and fairness." Vaccine risks were systematically understated or ignored. For example, the proposed guidelines state that "a few people will have a serious problem," but they do not mention that a "serious problem" could be permanent brain damage or death. The guidelines also reveal a selective use of scientific data, downplay the true rates of adverse reactions, and give inconsistent, incomplete, inaccurate, and potentially dangerous information regarding contraindications.[296]

The following quotes may shed some light on why the proposed guidelines were inadequate:

According to Barbara Loe Fisher, who also chairs the subcommittee on adverse reactions for the NVAC, "even though Congress gave the NVAC a dual mission: 'to achieve optimal prevention of human infectious disease through immunization' and 'to achieve optimal prevention against adverse reactions to vaccines,' I had observed that the majority of NVAC time was spent discussing how to promote vaccination. The equally important goal of identifying ways to prevent vaccine reactions appears to be a subject that causes discomfort among many committee members, is viewed as an obstacle to promoting vaccination, and is generally given little time or in-depth treatment."[297]

Fisher also notes that "not only is there a lack of concern about the subject of vaccine reactions on the part of some committee members, but there is a deliberate attempt to deny the reality of vaccine reactions, deaths and injuries... [Committee members need] to spend more time trying to find ways to solve problems associated with preventing vaccine reactions rather than trying to find ways to reword subcommittee reports to deny the existence of [children who were damaged or killed by a vaccine reaction]."[298]

In addition to all of the above, Drs. James Cherry and Edward Mortimer, two prominent doctors believed to be impartial advisors to HHS, the federal organization responsible for promoting vaccine safety guidelines, have been charged with failing to disclose conflicts of interest after it was discovered that they (and the research programs that support them) were paid by pertussis vaccine manufacturers over $800,000 in expert witness and consulting fees and research grants.[299]

Claims for Compensation: The general public is essentially unaware of the true number of people (mostly children) who have been permanently damaged or killed by the vaccines. According to Barbara L. Fisher, executive vice president of the National Vaccine Information Center (NVIC), figures from the U.S. Claims Court as of October 31, 1990, indicate that "...several thousand claims [for compensation from injuries or death caused by vaccines] have already been filed..."[300] In fact, *every year about 12,000 reports of adverse reactions to vaccines are made to the FDA* (data accessible only through the Freedom of Information Act). These figures include hospital visits, irreversible injuries, and hundreds of deaths.[301]

The general public is also essentially unaware of the amount of money awarded in these cases. In the last few years (by November 10, 1999), more than $1 BILLION had already been awarded for hundreds of injuries and deaths caused by mandated vaccines. Thousands of cases are still pending.[302] It should also be noted that awards were given for vaccine deaths and permanent injuries that included learning disabilities, seizure disorders, mental retardation, and paralysis. Many of the awards given for pertussis vaccine deaths *were initially misclassified as sudden infant death syndrome (SIDS).*[303]

Who pays for compensation? In order to pay for vaccine injuries or deaths occurring after October 1, 1988, Congress established a special tax on the sale of mandated vaccines. The amount of tax on each vaccine corresponds to the anticipated funds needed to pay for injuries or deaths resulting from that vaccine. This tax ranges from several dollars per dose for the DPT and MMR (measles, mumps, and rubella) vaccines, to several cents per dose for the polio and DT (diphtheria and tetanus) vaccines. This tax is passed on to consumers who are, in effect, paying insurance to cover the possibility that they may suffer a severe vaccine reaction.[304]

Are Vaccines Mandatory? Scare tactics, skewed statistics, and outright lies are often used by medical and health officials to intimidate wavering parents into vaccinating their children. For example, when recent television programs attacked the pertussis vaccine, the Maryland Health Department deceived the public by blaming a recent epidemic of whooping cough on the impact of these shows. However, when the former top virologist for the U.S. Division of Biological Standards, Dr. J. Anthony Morris, analyzed the original data provided by the Immunization Program Coordinator, he concluded the Maryland "epidemic" didn't exist. In only five of the 41 cases was there sufficient evidence to correctly diagnose whooping cough. And of these cases, each child had received from one to four doses of the pertussis vaccine.[305]

Again, in Placitas, New Mexico, recent headlines warned parents of a dangerous whooping cough epidemic in that town. But only three cases of whooping cough were discovered, two of them in siblings, all in children who were not "adequately" vaccinated.[306]

Many colleges are now requiring new students to be fully vaccinated as a prerequisite to admission.[307] And the Federal government has considered denying welfare and nutritional benefits to families who refuse vaccinations.[308] Meanwhile, doctors and school authorities tell parents that state laws and school regulations "absolutely require" their children to receive mandated vaccines. However, *most states provide waivers permitting parents to object to mandated vaccines* on personal, religious, or philosophical

Figure 12:
STATE of NEW MEXICO
VACCINE WAIVER FORM

New Mexico Department of Health
Public Health Division

CERTIFICATE OF
RELIGIOUS/CONSCIENTIOUS OBJECTION TO IMMUNIZATION

Please Print:

School _____ Parent/Guardian _____

Address _____ Address _____

_____ _____

Principal/Headperson _____

DIRECTIONS:

Please complete the following, giving your child's name, specifying your relationship to your child, and your address. Then, in the presence of a Notary Public, please sign and date the certificate and have it notarized.

In accordance with Section 24-5-3 A(3) NMSA 1978, I hereby certify that the administration of vaccine and other

immunizing agents to my child _____ , is contrary to my Religious beliefs, held either individually or jointly with others, and I therefore request that my child be exempted from the school immunization requirements of Section 24-5-2 NMSA 1978.

I UNDERSTAND THIS REQUEST IS SUBJECT TO THE APPROVAL OF THE NEW MEXICO DEPARTMENT OF HEALTH. I HAVE READ THE "COMPULSORY IMMUNIZATION REGULATIONS" AND UNDERSTAND THE RISK OF NON-IMMUNIZATION FOR MY CHILD. I UNDERSTAND THAT THIS CERTIFICATE IS VALID FOR A PERIOD NOT TO EXCEED NINE (9) MONTHS.

I swear that all the foregoing statements are true to the best of my information, knowledge and belief.

☐ Parent ☐ Guardian _____   _____
                                        Signature   _Date_

Subscribed and Sworn before me this _____ day of _____ , 19 ____ .

_____
NOTARY'S SIGNATURE AND SEAL

My Commission Expires: _____

· ·
(FOR PUBLIC HEALTH DIVISION USE ONLY)

☐ APPROVED ☐ DISAPPROVED _____   _____
                                           Authorized Signature   _Date_

grounds (Figure 12). A child may also be exempted if the parents can obtain a written statement from a doctor stating that the vaccine would be harmful to the child's health.

In spite of these waivers, parents have been charged with child abuse for not vaccinating their children, and they were hustled into court with the threat of losing custody of their loved ones. Court officials, social workers, and even foster parents have tried to take matters into their own hands by forcing injections on the children.[309] Ironically, parents have lost custody of their children and were accused of child abuse — "shaking baby syndrome" — when their babies had seizures or went into a coma following vaccinations.[310]

Authorities also argue that parents should vaccinate their children to protect society as a whole from epidemics. But if the vaccines offered true immunity only the unvaccinated would become ill.[311] Therefore, decisions that affect your child's health should not be forced upon you by so-called experts who are not even willing (nor able) to take responsibility for their actions.

For further information on vaccine regulations, call your State or County Health Department. ***Request a copy of the immunization laws.*** Or visit your regional law library. (State vaccine laws — and many other vaccine resources — are also available from New Atlantean Press: 505-983-1856.) If authorities are unrelenting in their efforts to intimidate and harass you, seek legal aid, or contact your local vaccine organization for support.

The Germ Theory: Some researchers argue that germs do not cause disease. If this is true, then the very foundations upon which vaccinations are built are flawed.[312] According to Dr. Antoine Bechamp, renowned scientist and bacteriologist, germs are an integral part of living cells. They remain dormant until the cell has completed its life cycle and begins to decay. Germs help to decompose the dying cell so that it may be eliminated from the body.[313] Dr. Robert Koch, another opponent of the germ theory, confirms Bechamp's explanation. He believes that if germs cause disease, then specific germs must a) be found in every case of the disease, and b) never be found apart from the disease. But germs do not conform to these requirements.[314]

According to the German bacteriologist, Guenther Enderlein, whose treatment techniques have been used in Europe for more than 40 years, certain bacteria can take on multiple forms during a single life cycle (pleomorphism). Some microbial forms that live in the human body are, under certain conditions, associated with many of the worst chronic diseases known to humankind. But when a person is healthy, these microbes are helpful to the body's immune system and live with the other cells in a symbiotic relationship. However, any severe change or deterioration of the body's internal environment — the "terrain" — due to poor nutrition or other factors, could cause the microbes to change into disease-causing forms as they pass through different stages of their life cycle. Simply put, "the germ is nothing, the terrain is everything."[315]

Louis Pasteur, the French chemist and bacteriologist who had the greatest influence on the course of medicine and the medical concept of disease, initially believed that all disease was caused by external microbes that invaded the body. He claimed that healthy tissues were germ-free. However, before Pasteur died, he retreated from this view and admitted that the internal environment was the key, but his earlier ideas endured.[316] Even Rudolph Virchow, German pathologist and founder of cellular medicine, stated: "If I could live my life over again, I would devote it to proving that germs seek their natural habitat — 'diseased' tissue — rather than being the cause of the 'diseased' tissue." And Dr. George White, MD, directly states that "if the germ theory were founded on facts, there would be no living being to read what's written."[317]

Natural Immunity: These researchers and others believe that a proper diet is essential to health. This means eating foods that are unrefined, organically grown, and preservative-free.[318,319] An improper diet overwhelms the system and leads to disease, for disease is the cleansing effort of the body to rid itself of an excess of toxins and waste material.[320] Adequate rest and sanitary living conditions are also integral to health. According to Harold Buttram, MD, when these requirements are met, "many diseases will pass as subclinical infections without acute illness, or if there is illness, it will be relatively mild."[321] Thus, natural immunity is best achieved by proper hygiene and wholesome living.

Research also indicates that breastfed newborns have healthier immune systems than babies that were bottle-fed.[322-324] And a panel of researchers in Chicago, headed by Roy Kupcinel, MD, reminded listeners that sugar weakens the immune system. Ingesting 100mg (less than .004 of an ounce) of sugar reduces the immune functions in the body by 50 percent within an hour.[325] Other studies confirm that excessive sugar consumption may increase the incidence of infections and reduce the body's ability to defend against disease.[326]

Finally, parents who are disenchanted with the allopathic or medical approach to illness might appreciate knowing that some doctors recommend homeopathy for the prevention and treatment of acute diseases.[327,328]

"The nutritionists of today will become the doctors of tomorrow." —Paavo Airola

SUMMARY AND CONCLUSION

A brief review of the data presented in this book indicates that:

1) Many of the vaccines were *not* the true cause of a decline in the incidence of the disease. Increased nutritional and sanitary measures probably deserve credit. Some diseases may also have their own evolutionary cycles; the virulent nature of the virgin disease is transformed into a tame illness as members of the population are exposed to it and gain "herd" immunity.

2) *None* of the vaccines can confer genuine immunity. Often the opposite is true; the vaccine *increases* the chance of contracting the disease. (Published "vaccine efficacy rates" are misleading. They are often evaluated by measuring blood antibody levels — not by comparing infection rates in vaccinated and unvaccinated persons.)[329]

3) All of the vaccines can produce side-effects. Reactions range from soreness at the injection site to brain damage and death.

4) The long-term effects of *all* vaccines are unknown. Particularly distressing are the implications that vaccines can be devastating to the young child's immature immune system. Studies were presented showing impaired health protection following injections. Lowered physical defenses may be responsible for a new breed of autoimmune diseases. Other studies showed damage to the brain and nervous system following shots — post-vaccinal encephalitis. This, in turn, causes large numbers of children to grow up with physical, mental and emotional disabilities of varying degrees. All of these conditions affect the individual, his or her family, and society as well.

5) Several of the vaccines can be especially dangerous. Nevertheless, the Medical-Industrial Complex continues to maintain its deceptive practice of disregarding vaccine reactions. In fact, medical officials recently suggested that they were justified in administering new and unproven vaccines by claiming it is unethical to withhold them!?[330] Meanwhile, creative propaganda on the merits of vaccinations remains a lucrative ploy. For example, the AMA admits that "adult vaccines need a gimmick." CDC physicians

suggest a catchy slogan, like "Vaccines are not just kid stuff."[331] Hollywood stars, such as Bill Cosby and Whoopi Goldberg, have been recruited as well. They have been seen and heard on TV and radio warning parents to "Vaccinate, before it's too late."[332] In England, the National Health Service pays a "bonus" to doctors with documented vaccination rates above specified percentages.[333] Of course, in the United States informal pressures and inducements to obey authority are not enough. Our medical policy-makers have lobbied for laws against freedom of choice. Their patterns of coercion and denial are notorious among the enlightened members of the population (parents who question vaccines), though sadly their awakenings may have cost them dearly — often the life or health of their own child.

Vaccinations are not the only basis for the unfortunate conditions noted throughout the text. Personal maladies and social ills have several causes. Nor are all members of the medical establishment callous and uncaring. Many are simply unaware of the true extent of damage being caused by vaccines. They sincerely believe that only good can come from being injected with foreign germs and toxic matter. But in a free country like the United States of America, no one should be compelled to submit to dangerous health practices against their will. Health and illness are personal experiences belonging to the people undergoing them. Nobody else has the right to dictate how they will be managed. That choice is the individual's alone, or belongs to the legitimate guardians of a dependent child.

Some mothers have long suspected that vaccines may not be appropriate for their children, but they worry about whether they can make the decision not to vaccinate and still be strong enough to face their pediatrician, family, and friends. Many fathers are also uneasy when questioning society and the status quo. They don't want to be considered "soft" on the vaccine issue. But the decision regarding whether or not to vaccinate is the parent's alone. It must not be based upon irrational factors. Instead, this choice should be made only after examining credible evidence from several sources. In addition, critical thinking should be exercised when interpreting information. I encourage parents to substantiate all of the references in this book, and to research this topic even further if questions still remain. As parents, you are entitled to — and responsible for obtaining — the facts regarding the benefits and risks of vaccinating your children.

"Health is not a condition of matter, but of Mind." —Mary Baker Eddy

Notes

1. William A. R. Thomson, *Black's Medical Dictionary* (Totawa, NJ: Barnes & Noble Books, 1987), p. 716.

2. *World Book Encyclopedia,* Volume 11 (1989), p. 89.

3. W. A. Volk and M. F. Wheeler, *Basic Microbiology, 4th ed.* (Philadelphia, PA: J.B. Lippincott Co., 1980), p. 455.

4. M. Burnet and D. White, *The Natural History of Infectious Disease* (New York, NY: Cambridge University Press, 1972), p. 16.

5. Richard Moskowitz, MD, "Immunizations: The Other Side," *Mothering* (Spring 1984), p. 36.

6. Robert Mendelsohn MD, *How To Raise A Healthy Child...In Spite of Your Doctor* (Chicago: Contemporary Books, 1984), p. 228.

7. Michael Alderson, *International Mortality Statistics* (Washington, DC: Facts on File, 1981), pp. 177-178.

8. See Note 6, pp. 210; 228.

9. Hannah Allen, *Don't Get Stuck: The Case Against Vaccinations...,* (Oldsmar, FL: Natural Hygiene Press, 1985), p. 146. Also see Note 10, p. 140.

10. Eleanor McBean, *The Poisoned Needle,* (Mokelumne Hill, CA: Health Research, 1974), p. 142.

11. Ibid., p. 144

12. Ibid., pp. 142-145.

13. Hearings before the Committee on Interstate and Foreign Commerce, House of Rep., 87th Congress, 2nd Session on HR 10541, May '62, pp. 94-112.

14. Christopher Kent, DC, Ph.D., "Drugs, Bugs, and Shots in the Dark," *Health Freedom News,* (January 1983), p. 26.

15. M. Beddow Bayly, *The Case Against Vaccination,* (York Road, London: William H. Taylor & Sons, Ltd., Printers, June 1936), p. 4.

16. *Washington Post,* (September 24, 1976).

17. American Academy of Pediatrics, *Report of the Committee on Infectious Diseases: 1986,* (Elk Grove Village, IL: AAP), pp. 284-285.

18. Peter. M. Strebel, et al., "Epidemiology of Poliomyelitis in the U.S. One Decade after the Last Reported Case of Indigenous Wild Virus Associated Disease," *Clinical Infectious Diseases,* (CDC, February 1992), pp. 568-79.

19. *20th Immunization Conference Proceedings, Dallas, Texas, May 6-9, 1985,* (U.S. Department of Health and Human Services, October 1985), p. 85.

20. See Note 18.

21. Daniel Chasan, "The Polio Paradox," *Science* (April 1986), p. 39.

22. Benjamin P. Sandler, MD, *Diet Prevents Polio,* (The Lee Foundation for Nutritional Research, 1951). Also see Note 10, pp. 116-118; 146.

23. Ibid., p. 146.

24. See Note 22, p. 43.

25. See Note 10, p. 146.

26. See Note 5, p. 35.

27. *Morbidity and Mortality Weekly Report Summary*, (U.S. Govt. 1993).

28. See Note 7, pp. 161-162.

29. "A Mother's Research on Immunizations," *Mothering* (Fall '79), p. 76.

30. See Note 5, p. 35.

31. Eleanor McBean, Ph.D., *Vaccinations Do Not Protect,* (Manachaca, TX: Health Excellence Systems, 1991), p. 8.

32. See Note 10, p. 19.

33. See Note 31.

34. *November 20-21, 1975, Minutes of the 15th meeting of the Panel of Review of Bacterial Vaccines and Toxoids with Standards and Potency,* (presented by the Bureau of Biologics and the Food and Drug Administration).

35. See Note 6, p. 223.
36. See Note 5, p. 34.
37. Ibid.
38. See Note 6, pp. 214-215.
39. See Note 5, p. 34.
40. See Note 6, pp. 214-215.
41. See Note 6. p. 215.
42. See Note 7, pp. 182-183.
43. See Note 6, p. 216.
44. J. Cherry, "The New Epidemiology of Measles and Rubella," *Hospital Practice,* (July 1980), p. 49.
45. *World Book Encyclopedia,* Volume 13 (1989), p. 345.
46. *National Health Federation Bulletin,* (Nov. '69). Also see Note 6, p. 216.
47. *FDA Workshop to Review Warnings, Use Instructions, and Precautionary Information [on Vaccines],* (Rockland, Maryland, Sept. 18, 1992), p. 27.
48. John A. Frank, Jr., MD, et al., "Measles Elimination — Final Impediments," *20th Immunization Conference Proceedings, May 6-9, 1985,* p. 21.
49. *Morbidity and Mortality Weekly Report,* (U.S. Govt., June 6, 1986).
50. *Morbidity and Mortality Weekly Report,* (U.S. Govt., Dec. 29, 1989).
51. See Note 6, p. 215.
52. N. P. Thompson, et al. "Is Measles Vaccine a Risk Factor for Inflammatory Bowel Disease?" *Lancet,* (April 29, 1995), pp. 1071 +.
53. M. Rizzetto, et al., *J. of Infectious Diseases* (January 1982), pp. 18-22.
54. "Immunizations and Informed Consent," *Mothering* (Winter '83), p. 41; *Measles, Mumps, & Rubella: What You Need to Know,* (CDC, '91) p. 1.
55. Daniel Q. Haney, "Wave of Infant Measles Stems From '60s Vaccinations," *Albuquerque Journal,* (November 23, 1992), p. B3.
56. Gerald T. Keusch, "Vitamin A Supplements — Too Good Not to Be True," *New England Journal of Medicine,* (October 4, 1990), pp. 985-987.
57. *Vaccine Injury Compensation.* Hearings Before the Subcommittee on Health & the Environment; 98th Congress, 2nd Session, (Dec. 19, 1984), p. 110.
58. See Note 6, p. 217.
59. Robert S. Mendelsohn, MD, *But Doctor, About That Shot...The Risks of Immunizations and How to Avoid Them,* (Evanston, IL: The People's Doctor Newsletter, Inc., 1988), p. 4.
60. Ibid., p. 12.
61. Ibid., p. 31.
62. Dr. B. Allan, *Australian J. of Medical Technology. 4,* (1973), pp. 26-27.
63. See Note 6, p. 218.
64. Ibid.
65. M. Lawless, et al., "Rubella Susceptibility in Sixth-Graders," *Pediatrics,* 65 (June 1980), pp. 1086-1089.
66. Dr. Allen B. Allen, "Is RA27/3 a Cause of Chronic Fatigue?" *Medical Hypothesis,* 27 (1988), pp. 217-220.
67. Dr. A.D. Lieberman, "The Role of the Rubella Virus in the Chronic Fatigue Syndrome," *Clinical Ecology,* Vol. 7, No. 3, pp. 51-54.
68. See Note 6, pp. 217-218.
69. See Note 9, p. 144.
70. *Vaccine Reaction Report,* (Vienna, VA: National Vaccine Information Center, November 25, 1991), pp. 23-24.
71. "Rubella Shots for Hospital Employees," *The Doctor's People: A Medical Newsletter for Consumers,* (Evanston, IL, August 1991), pp. 1-2.
72. "Rubella Vaccine and Susceptible Hospital Employees: Poor Physician Participation," *Journal of the American Medical Association,* (February 20, 1981).
73. See Note 5, p. 35.
74. See Notes 6, p. 213; 47, pp. 29-30.
75. See Note 6, p. 214.
76. Ibid., pp. 213-214.
77. Ibid., p. 214.
78. Jane McDonald, et al., "Clinical and Epidemiological Features of Mumps Meningo-encephalitis and Possible Vaccine-Related Disease," *Pediatric Infectious Disease Journal,* (November 1989), pp. 751-754.
79. R. Moskowitz. In a correction in an unpublished version of this article.
80. R. Moskowitz, "Unvaccinated Children," *Mothering* (Winter '87), p. 36.
81. "A Mother Researches Immunization," *Mothering* (Summer '80), p. 41.

82. See Note 5, p. 35.
83. Edward Mortimer, "Immunization Against Infectious Disease," *Science*, Volume 200, (May 26, 1978), p. 905.
84. See Note 59, p. 41.
85. Ibid.
86. Isaac Golden, Ph.D., *Vaccination? A Review of Risks and Alternatives*, (Geelong, Victoria, Australia: Arum Healing Centre, 1991), p. 31.
87. See Note 59, p. 41.
88. Ibid., p. 71.
89. See Note 9, p. 167.
90. M. Eibl, MD, et al., "Abnormal T-Lymphocyte Subpopulations in Healthy Subjects after Tetanus Booster Immunizations," *New England Journal of Medicine*, Vol. 310, (Nov. 26, 1981), pp. 1307-1313.
91. Harold E. Buttram, MD and John Chriss Hoffman, "Bringing Vaccines Into Perspective," *Mothering*, (Winter 1985), p. 30.
92. See Note 5.
93. See Note 6, p. 219.
94. See Note 5.
95. See Note 7, pp. 164-165.
96. S. A. Halperin, et al., "Persistence of Pertussis in an Immunized Population: Results of the Nova Scotia Enhanced Pertussis Surveillance Program," *Journal of Pediatrics* (Nov. 1989), pp. 686-693.
97. M. E. Pichichero, et al., "Diphtheria-Pertussis-Tetanus Vaccine: Reactogenicity of Commercial Products," *Pediatrics* (Feb. 1979), pp. 256-260.
98. *Whooping Cough, the DPT Vaccine and Reducing Vaccine Reactions* (Vienna, VA., National Vaccine Information Center 1989), p. 3.
99. See Note 19, pp. 83-84.
100. *Vaccine Bulletin* (February 1987), p. 11.
101. D. C. Christie, et al., "The 1993 Epidemic of Pertussis in Cincinnati: Resurgence of Disease in a Highly Immunized Population of Children," *New England Journal of Medicine* (July 7, 1994), pp. 16-20.
102. *Physicians' Desk Reference*, (Montvale, NJ: Medical Economics Data Production, 1995). Also see *Physicians' GenRx*, (NY: Data Pharmaceutica, 1993).
103. Drs. Cherry, Brunell, et al., "Report of the Task Force on Pertussis and Pertussis Immunization," *Pediatrics*, 81:6, pt. 2 (June 1988), p. 943.
104. Harris L. Coulter, *Vaccination, Social Violence, and Criminality: Medical Assault on the American Brain*, (Berkeley, CA: North Atlantic, 1990), p. xiv.
105. Harris L. Coulter and Barbara Loe Fisher, *A Shot in the Dark: Why the P in DPT Vaccination May be Hazardous to Your Child's Health*, (Garden City Park, NY: Avery Publishing Group, 1991), pp. 13-14.
106. Ibid., p. 11.
107. Ibid., pp. 32-34. Also see Note 99, pp. 10-16; Note 6, pp. 221-222.
108. *Immunization: Survey of Recent Research*, (United States Department of Health and Human Services, April 1983), p. 76.
109. "Nature and the Rates of Adverse Reactions Associated with DTP and DT Immunizations...," *Pediatrics*, Volume 68, No. 5 (Nov 1981), pp. 650-59.
110. Michel Odent, et al., "Pertussis Vaccination and Asthma: Is There a Link?" *J. of the American Medical Association*, (Aug 24/31, 1994), pp. 592-3.
111. J. M. Fine and L. C. Chen, "Confounding in studies of adverse reactions to vaccines," *American Journal of Epidemiology*, 136, (1992), pp. 121-35.
112. See Note 105, p. 51.
113. Dr. Viera Scheibnerova and Leif Karlsson, *Association Between Non-Specific Stress Syndrome, DPT Injections, and Cot Death*, (2nd Immunization Conference, Canberra, Australia, May 27-29, 1991).
114. W. C. Torch, "Diphtheria-pertussis-tetanus (DPT) immunization: A potential cause of the sudden infant death syndrome (SIDS)," (Amer. Academy of Neurology, 34th Annual Meeting, Apr 25 - May 1, 1982), *Neurology* 32(4), pt. 2.
115. *Vaccine Injury Compensation.* Hearing Before the Committee on Labor and Human Resources; 98th Congress, 2nd Session, (May 3, 1984), pp. 63-67.
116. S.732, S.733, H.R.1640; 103rd Congress, 1st Session, (April 1, '93).
117. Carl Tant, *Awesome Green*, (Angleton, TX: Biotech Pub., 1994), pp. 108-115. Also: H.R. 78, 103rd Congress, 1st Session: A Bill, (Jan. 5, 1993).
118. Richard Moskowitz, MD, "Vaccination: A Sacrament of Modern Medicine," *Mothering*, (Spring 1992), p. 53.
119. Richard Leviton, "A Shot in the Dark," *Yoga Journal*, (May/June,

1992), p. 128.
120. See Note 105, pp. 208-210; *AAP News Release,* (April 15, 1992).
121. See Note 59, p. 81.
122. See Note 105, pp. 210-212.
123. "Pertussis Vaccines: Trials and Tribulations," *JAMA,* (April 8, 1988).
124. Marian Tompson; see Note 59, p. 96.
125. R. Weiss, "Meningitis Vaccine Stirs Controversy," *Science News,* Volume 132, (October 24, 1987), p. 260.
126. Sydney S. Gellis, MD, ed., *Pediatric Notes: The Weekly Pediatric Commentary,* Volume 11:2, (January 15, 1987).
127. Robert S. Mendelsohn, MD, "New Vaccine to Combat Day Care Infections," *The People's Doctor Newsletter,* (Volume 9, No. 11), p. 5. (Figures reported by Dr. Stephen L. Coeni of the Centers for Disease Control).
128. "'Meningitis' Vaccine is Really Not...," *Pediatric Patter,* (Aug. 1986).
129. See Note 59, p. 5.
130. L. H. Harrison, et al, "Case-control efficacy study of the polysaccharide (Hib) vaccine," *Abstracts of the 27th ICAAC, New York,* (1987), No. 319.
131. "Policy Statement: Haemophilus b Polysaccharide Vaccine (HbPV)," *American Academy of Pediatrics (AAP) News,* (November 1987), p. 7.
132. See Note 59, p. 87.
133. "Meningitis Risk Seen from Use of Vaccine," *St. Paul Pioneer Press Dispatch,* (April 21, 1987).
134. Ibid.
135. See Note 59, p. 87.
136. Ibid., p. 88.
137. See Note 125.
138. See Note 131.
139. See Note 126.
140. See Note 127.
141. C. E. Emery Jr., "In the Pub. Health," *Providence J. Bull.,* (Dec. '86).
142. See Note 125.
143. "Updates: Vaccine Use Extended to Infants," *FDA Consumer,* (January-February 1991), p. 2.
144. See Notes 125, 143.
145. See Note 125.
146. Alter, M.J., Hadler, S.C., et al. "The changing epidemiology of hepatitis B in the U.S." *J. of the American Medical Assoc.* 1990; 263: pp. 1218-1222.
147. Institute of Medicine, *Adverse Events Associated with Childhood Vaccines: Evidence Bearing on Causality.* Wash., DC: National Acad. Press, 1994.
148. Robert S. Mendelsohn, MD, "The Drive to Immunize Adults is On," *Herald of Holistic Health Newsletter,* (September-October, 1985), p. 2.
149. Freed, G.L., et al. "Family physician acceptance of universal hepatitis B immunization of infants." *Journal of Family Practice* 1993; 36: pp. 153-157.
150. NVIC Press Release on Hepatitis B (January 27, 1999), p. 3.
151. *Hepatitis B Vaccines: What You Should Know,* (New Atlantean, 1998)
152. See Note 59, p. 3.
153. See Note 59, pp. 3-4, and Note 110, p. 54.
154. See Note 148.
155. See Note 59, p. 75.
156. Randall Neustaedter, *The Vaccine Guide,* (North Atlantic, '96): 182-5.
157. "Chicken Pox Conundrum," *Time* (July 19,1993), p. 53.
158. See Note 10, pp. 12-20.
159. Ibid., p. 13.
160. Ibid., p. 16.
161. See Note 31, p. 26.
162. See Note 10, p. 13.
163. Ibid.
164. Ibid., p. 103.
165. See Note 31, p. 8.
166. See Note 10, p. 13.
167. Ibid., p. 60.
168. Ibid., p. 40
169. Ibid., p. 64.
170. Ibid., pp. 12-13.
171. See Note 59, p. 90.

172. See Note 10, pp. 28-29, 66.
173. Dr. Richard Moskowitz, "Immunizations: A Dissenting View," *Dissent in Medicine — Nine Doctors Speak Out,* (Contemporary Books, '85), pp. 133-166.
174. See Note 5, pp. 33-34.
175. Harold E. Buttram, MD and J. C. Hoffman, *Vaccinations and Immune Malfunctions,* (Humanitarian Publishing Co., 1982), p. 47.
176. Walene James, *Immunization: The Reality Behind the Myth,* (Bergin & Garvey, 1988), pp. 14-15.
177. Drs. Kalokerinos and Dettman, "A Supportive Submission," *The Dangers of Immunisation,* (Warburton, Victoria, Australia: Biological Research Institute, 1979), p. 49.
178. See Note 91, p. 32.
179. Ibid.
180. Richard Moskowitz, MD, *The Case Against Immunizations,* (Washington, DC: The National Center for Homeopathy, 1983), p. 15.
181. See Note 176, pp. 15-16.
182. Ibid., pp. 16-17.
183. *World Medicine,* (London: Clareville House, Sept. 22, '71), pp. 69-72.
184. See Note 176, p. 10.
185. H. E. Buttram, MD, "Live Virus Vaccines and Genetic Mutation," *Health Consciousness,* (April 1990), pp. 44-45.
186. G. Blanck, et al, "Multiple Insertions and Tandem Repeats of Origin-Mins Simian Virus 40 DNA in Transformed Rat and Mouse Cells," *Journal of Virology,* (May 1988), pp. 1520-1523.
187. S. Kumar, et al, "Effects of Serial Passage of Autographa Californiica Nuclear Polyhedrosis Virus in Cell Culture," *Virus Research,* 7 ('87), pp. 335-349.
188. See Note 185, p. 44.
189. J. Lederberg, *Science,* (October 20, 1967), p. 313.
190. See Note 185, p. 44.
191. T.J. Crow, "Is Schizophrenia an Infectious Disease?" *Lancet,* (1983), 1:8317, pp. 173-175.
192. Halonen, et al, "Antibody Levels to HSV-1, Measles, and Rubella Virus in Psychiatric Patients," *British Journal of Psychiatry,* 125 (1974), pp. 461-465.
193. D. Steinberg, et al, "Influenza Infection Causing Manic Psychosis," *British Journal of Psychiatry,* 120 (1972), pp. 531-535.
194. P.V. Morozov, ed., "Research on the Viral Hypothesis of Mental Disorders," *Advances in Biological Psychiatry,* Volume 12, (New York: S. Karger, 1983), pp. 52-75.
195. R. McGuire, "Brain Autoantibodies in 33% of Schizophrenics," *Medical Tribune,* (July 14, 1988), p. 6.
196. See Note 185, p. 45.
197. B.L. Horvath, et al., "Excretion of SV-40 virus after oral administration of contaminated polio vaccine," *Acta Microbiologica Hungary,* 11, pp. 271-275.
198. Arthur Snider, "Near Disaster with Salk Vaccine," *Sci. Digest,* (1963).
199. "Division of Biologics Standards: The Boat That Never Rocked," *Science,* (March 17, 1972).
200. William Bennett, *The Atlantic Monthly,* (Harvard University Press: February, 1976).
201. Eva Lee Snead, MD, "AIDS — Immunization Related Syndrome," *Health Freedom News,* (July 1987), p. 1
202. William Campbell Douglass, MD, "WHO Murdered Africa," *Health Freedom News,* (September 1987), p. 42.
203. Walter S. Kyle, "Simian retroviruses, poliovaccine, and origin of AIDS," *Lancet,* (March 7, 1992), pp. 600-601.
204. Tom Curtis, "The Origin of AIDS: A Startling New Theory Attempts to Answer the Question 'Was it an Act of God or an Act of Man,'" *Rolling Stone,* (March 19, 1992), pp. 54+.
205. Ibid., p. 57. Also see Notes 59, pp. 73, 79; 176, p. 101.
206. See Note 204, pp. 58-59.
207. Ibid., pp. 59-60, 108.
208. Tom Curtis, "Expert says test vaccine," *The Houston Post,* (March 22, 1992), p. A-21.
209. Ibid.
210. See Note 203.
211. *London Times,* (May 11, 1987), p. 1.

212. Ibid.
213. Department of Defense Appropriations for 1970: Hearings before a Subcommittee of the Committee on Appropriations, House of Representatives, Ninety-First Congress, First Session, H.B. 15090, July 1, 1969.
214. See Note 202, p. 19.
215. Allison, et al., "Virus-associated immunopathology," *Bulletin of the World Health Organization*, Volume 47, (1972), p. 259.
216. See Notes 202, p. 19; 204, p. 106.
217. *Strecker Report,* (Northglenn, CO: Triputic, Inc.). See Note 202, p. 26.
218. See Note 211.
219. "400,000 Human Guinea Pigs in the Persian Gulf: Illegal Experiments with Unapproved Drugs on American Troops," *Health Letter,* (Washington, DC: Public Citizen Health Research Group, February 12, 1991), p. 1.
220. See Note 202. Also see Note 217, *Strecker Report.*
221. See Note 204, p. 106.
222. Ibid., p. 108.
223. See Note 119, pp. 112-114.
224. See Note 104, pp. xiii-xiv; Chapters 1-5.
225. R. Bannister, *Brain's Clinical Neurology,* Fifth Edition, (Oxford: University Press, 1978), p. 409.
226. See Note 104.
227. Ibid., p. 103.
228. H.H. Merritt, *Textbook of Neurology,* Sixth Edition, (Philadelphia, PA: Lea and Febiger, 1979), p. 104.
229. Josephine B. Neal, *Encephalitis: A Clinical Study,* (New York: Grune and Stratton, 1942), pp. 378-379.
230. See Note 228, pp. 102-103.
231. See Note 228.
232. See Note 229.
233. Anna Lisa Annell, "Pertussis in Infancy — A Cause of Behavioral Disorders in Children," *Acta Societatis Medicorum Upsaliensis,* XVIII, Supplement 1, (1953), pp. 17, 33.
234. A.B. Baker, "The Central Nervous System in Infectious Diseases of Childhood," *Postgraduate Medicine,* 5, (1949), p. 11.
235. Lurie, et al, "Late Results Noted in Children Presenting Post-Encephalitic Behavior," *American Journal of Psychiatry,* 104, (1947), p. 178.
236. Frank R. Ford, *Diseases of the Nervous System in Infancy, Childhood, and Adolescence,* (Springfield: C.C. Thomas, 1937), p. 349.
237. See Note 104, pp. 120-121.
238. Leo Kanner, "Autistic Disturbances of Affective Content," *The Nervous Child II,* (1942-1943), p. 250.
239. American Psychiatric Association, *Diagnostic and Statistical Manual of Mental Disorders,* Third Edition, Revised, (Washington, DC, 1987), pp. 36-37.
240. S. Wakabayashi, "The Present Status of an Early Infantile Autism First Reported in Japan 30 Years Ago," *Nagoya Medical Journal,* 46, (1984), pp. 35 +.
241. See Note 104, p. 50.
242. Ibid.
243. Leo Kanner, "To What Extent is Early Infantile Autism Determined by Constitutional Inadequacies?" *Genetics and the Inheritance of Integrated Neurological and Psychiatric Patterns,* (Baltimore: Williams and Wilkins, 1954), p. 382.
244. Leo Kanner, et al., "Early Infantile Autism: 1943-1955," *Psychiatric Research Reports,* 7, (1957), p. 62.
245. Leo Kanner, "Early Infantile Autism," *Journal of Pediatrics,* 25, (1944), p. 217.
246. C. Gillberg and H. Schaumann, "Social Class and Infantile Autism," *Journal of Autism,* 12:3, (1982), p. 223.
247. See Note 104, pp. 52-53.
248. D.M. Ross and S.A. Ross, *Hyperactivity: Research, Theory, and Action,* (New York: John Wiley, 1982).
249. V.S. Cowart, "Attention-Deficit Hyperactivity Disorder: Physicians Helping Parents Pay More Heed," *Journal of American Medical Association,* 259:18, (May 13, 1988), p. 2647.
250. Kathleen Long and D.V. Queen, "Detection and Treatment of Emotionally Disturbed Children in Public Schools: Problems and Theoretical Perspectives," *Journal of Clinical Psychology,* 40:1, (January 1984), p. 378.

251. See Note 249.
252. Jane M. Healy, Ph.D., *Endangered Minds: Why Our Children Don't Think,* (New York: Simon & Schuster, Inc., 1990), pp. 13-15.
253. Ibid.
254. Ibid., pp. 17-18.
255. Ibid., pp. 27-35.
256. See Note 104, pp. 61-62.
257. Ibid., p. 112.
258. "Vaccine Fund Needs Booster Shot," *Common Cause Magazine,* (May/June, 1991), p. 10.
259. See Note 104, p. 113.
260. Ibid., p. 112.
261. Ibid., p. 113.
262. "Vaccine-injured Girl Gets $2.4 Million," *Tampa Tribune,* (May 16, 1990), p. 1B.
263. "When Vaccines Backfire," *Florida Today,* (July 30, 1990), p. 1-2A.
264. "Congress Votes Help to Youngster Hurt by Vaccine," *Tucson Citizen,* (May 9, 1990), p. 1-2A.
265. See Note 104, pp. 179-181.
266. E.D. Bond and K.E. Appel, *The Treatment of Behavior Disorders Following Encephalitis,* (New York: The Commonwealth Fund, 1931), p. 14-15.
267. Frank A. Elliott, "Biological Roots of Violence," *Proceedings of the American Philosophical Society,* 127:2 (1983), pp. 84-93.
268. *The New York Times,* (December 5, 1987), p. B1.
269. Bernard Rimland and G.E. Larson, "The Manpower Quality Decline: An Ecological Perspective," *Armed Forces and Society,* 8:1, (Fall 1981), p. 56.
270. See Note 104, pp. 186-187.
271. Dorothy Lewis, ed., *Vulnerabilities to Delinquency,* (New York: SP Medical and Scientific Books, 1981), p. 28.
272. H.E. Hollander and F.D. Turner, "Characteristics of Incarcerated Delinquents: Relationship Between Development Disorders, Environmental and Family Factors, and Patterns of Offense and Recidivism," *Journal of American Child Psychiatry,* 24:1, (1985), p. 225.
273. See Note 249.
274. K.E. Moyer, *The Psychobiology of Aggression,* (New York: Harper and Row, 1976), p. 36.
275. *Plan for a Nationwide Action on Epilepsy,* (Commission for the Control of Epilepsy, 1977), Volume 2, part 1, p. 822. (Unpublished material cited in Note 104, pp. 197-198.)
276. *The New York Times,* (September 17, 1985), p. C1 +.
277. See Note 252, p. 140.
278. T.I. Lidsky, et al, "Are Movement Disorders the Most Serious Side Effects of Maintenance Therapy with Antipsychotic Drugs?" *Biological Psychiatry,* 16:12, (1981), pp. 1189-1194.
279. V.S. Cowart, "The Ritalin Controversy: What's Made This Drug's Opponents Hyperactive?" *Journal of the American Medical Association,* 259:17, (May 6, 1988), p. 2522.
280. K.L. Workman-Daniels, et al., "Childhood Problem Behavior and Neuropsychological Functioning in Persons at Risk for Alcoholism," *Journal of Studies on Alcoholism,* Volume 48:3, (1987), pp. 187-193.
281. Irwin G. Sarason and Barbara R. Sarason, *Abnormal Psychology,* Sixth Edition, (Englewood Cliffs, NJ: Prentice Hall, 1989), p. 433.
282. The National Childhood Vaccine Injury Act of 1986, Public Law 99-660, *The Compensation System and How it Works.* (National Vaccine Information Center, Vienna, VA., 1990), pp. 1-7.
283. See Note 45.
284. See Note 99., pp. 7-10.
285. In a Sept. 16, 1990 letter written by Barbara Loe Fisher, to Donald A. Henderson, chairman of the National Vaccine Advisory Committee, p. 3.
286. *NVIC Mini News.* (National Vaccine Information Center, Vienna, VA., November 1990), p. 3.
287. See Note 70, pp. 4-15.
288. See Note 105, pp. 176-177.
289. Herbert M. Shelton, ND, *Vaccine and Serum Evils,* (San Antonio, TX: Dr. Shelton's Health School, 1966), p. 34.

290. See Note 99, pp. 8-10.

291. Barkin and Pichichero, "Diphtheria-pertussis-tetanus vaccine: Reactogenicity of commercial products," *Pediatrics,* 63:2, (Feb. 2, '79), pp. 256-260.

292. See Note 105, pp. 55-56.

293. See Note 176, p. 19.

294. *Vaccine Safety Committee Proceedings,* (Institute of Medicine, National Academy of Sciences, Washington, DC, May 11, 1992), pp. 93-105.

295. *NVIC Mini News.* (NVIC, Vienna, VA., March 1991), p. 1.

296. In a February 25, 1991 letter written by Jeffrey H. Schwartz of NVIC, to Walter A. Orenstein, M.D., director of the Division of Immunization, CDC, with accompanying *Comments on Proposed Vaccine Information Materials;* in a March 13, 1991 letter to Dr. Claire Broome of the CDC, with accompanying appendices.

297. See Note 285, p. 1.

298. Ibid., p. 2.

299. In a May 8, 1991 letter written by Jeffrey H. Schwartz of NVIC, to Louis M. Sullivan, secretary of the Department of Health and Human Services; in a May 9, 1991 press release issued by NVIC.

300. See Note 286, p. 1.

301. Vaccine Adverse Event Reporting System (VAERS), Rockville, MD.

302. National Vaccine Injury Compensation Program, "Monthly Statistics Report." (Awards Paid through November 10, 1999.)

303. See Note 286, p. 2.

304. See Note 282, p. 8.

305. See Note 59, p. 34.

306. Reprint from a newspaper article. (In a handout by the National Vaccine Information Center, Vienna, VA.)

307. "Campus Ills," *Time,* (March 11, '85), p. 66. Also see Note 52, p. 22.

308. Philip, J. Hilts, "U.S. Vaccine Plan Uses Welfare Offices," *New York Times,* (March 17, 1991), p. 26.

309. See Note 176, pp. 131-146.

310. See Note 70, pp. 20-21.

311. See Note 80, p. 34.

312. Dr. Paavo Airola, "Immunization: A New Look," *Everywoman's Book,* (Phoenix, AZ: Health Plus, 1979), pp. 271-285.

313. See Notes 10, p. 9; 31, pp. 13-14.

314. E. Douglas Hume, *Bechamp or Pasteur,* (Mokelumne Hill, CA: Health Research, 1989). Abridged reprint by Health Research. Also see Note 313.

315. Michael Sheehan, "Was Pasteur Wrong?," *Natural Health,* (Jan/Feb 1992), pp. 41-44.

316. Ibid.

317. See Note 314.

318. See Notes 29, p. 79; 312, pp. 285-287.

319. See Note 176, pp. 195-197. (Appendix A: Keys to a Healthy Immune System — A Holistic Approach).

320. See Note 10, p. 9.

321. See Note, 91, p. 31.

322. R. Weiss, "Breastmilk May Stimulate Immunity," *Science News,* (March 26, 1988), p. 196.

323. Lindsey Grossman, "Breastfeeding Healthier Babies," *USA Today,* (August 1988), p. 4.

324. Allan Cunningham, MD, "Breastfeeding and Health," *The Compleat Mother,* (Summer 1987), p. 36.

325. Marian Tompson; see Note 59, p. 96.

326. William Manahan, MD, *Eat For Health,* (Tiburon, CA: H.J. Kramer, Inc., 1988), pp. 60-76.

327. See Note 80, pp. 35-38.

328. Dr. Dorothy Shepherd, *Homeopathy in Epidemic Diseases,* (United Kingdom: Health Sciences Press, 1967).

329. See Note 47, pp. 54-55.

330. Ibid., pp. 163-165.

331. "Is a 'Gimmick' the Answer?," *AMA News,* (Feb. 1, 1985), pp. 1 +.

332. "Stars Say 'Get Your Shots!,'" *Weekly Reader,* (Feb. 21, 1992), p. 1.

333. Richard Moskowitz, MD, "Vaccination: A Sacrament of Modern Medicine." Presented in a speech at the Annual Conference of the Society of Homeopaths, (Manchester, England, September 1991).

More Vaccine Books

By Neil Z. Miller

Vaccine Reactions: The Hidden Epidemic

NEW! This comprehensive treatise on vaccine damage (and how to protect your children) includes recent Congressional hearings on vaccines, and the latest studies linking the shots to autism, diabetes, multiple sclerosis, and lots more. Expected availability: Fall 2001. Reserve your copy today.

Immunization Theory vs. Reality

Code#: ITH $12.95   160 pages   © 1999, updated   1-881217-12-4

* A profound exposé of the vaccine industry.
* Contains the most compelling, **up-to-date studies** available.
* Lists vaccine ingredients and **medical ploys** used to hoodwink parents.
* Reveals the link between **experimental shots** and Gulf War Syndrome.
* Clarifies immune system development and **health options.**
* Offers **complete documentation** and **solutions** to this dilemma.

"If anything should be compulsory in the USA, it is the reading of this book by every politician, medical doctor, parent, and citizen."
—Dr. Viera Scheibner

Immunizations: The People Speak!

Code#: ITP $8.95   80 pages   © 1998, updated   1-881217-16-7

* **Riveting transcripts** of radio and TV interviews given by the author.
* A candid presentation of **crucial vaccine data.**
* Includes safety issues, legal rights, personal stories, and options.

"As a pediatric nurse, and as a concerned parent, I know what a complex issue this is. Thank you, Mr. Miller; great job!"
—Jane Watson, RN

---

* * * To Order These Books * * *

Individuals: Send the total money due, plus 7% shipping ($3.50 minimum), to: *New Atlantean Press*, PO Box 9638-925, Santa Fe, NM 87504. Bookstores: Order from your favorite wholesaler or distributor.

PURCHASING INFORMATION

Additional copies of **Vaccines: Are They *Really* Safe and Effective?** (ISBN: 1-881217-10-8), may be obtained from *New Atlantean Press*. Call <u>505-983-1856</u>. Or send $8.95 (in U.S. funds), plus $3.50 shipping, to:

New Atlantean Press
PO Box 9638-925
Santa Fe, NM 87504
505-983-1856 (Telephone & Fax)

Immunization Theory vs. Reality: Exposé on Vaccinations (160p., $12.95, ISBN: 1-881217-12-4) and **Immunizations: The People Speak! Questions, Comments, and Concerns About Vaccinations** (80p. $8.95, ISBN: 1-881217-16-7), both by Neil Z. Miller, may also be purchased from *New Atlantean Press*. Please add shipping charges. These books are also available at many fine book and health food stores.

Bookstores and Retail Buyers: Order from Baker & Taylor, Bookpeople, Ingram, Midpoint Trade Books, New Leaf, Nutri-Books (T-974), or from New Atlantean Press. Libraries may order from their favorite wholesaler.

Chiropractors, Homeopaths, Midwives, Naturopaths, Pediatricians, Vaccine Organizations, and other Non-Storefront Buyers: Take a 40% discount with the purchase of 5 or more copies (multiply the total cost of purchases x .60). Please add 7% ($3.50 minimum) for shipping.

Shipping: Please add 7% ($3.50 minimum) for shipping. Allow one to three weeks for your order to arrive, or include $2.50 extra for priority air mail shipping. Foreign orders must include 9% ($4.00 minimum) for shipping; $6 each for air mail. Checks must be drawn on a U.S. bank, or send a Postal Money Order in U.S. funds. **Sales Tax:** Please add 6% for books shipped to New Mexico addresses.

FREE CATALOG: *New Atlantean Press* offers the world's largest selection of vaccine information, including up-to-date vaccination laws, vaccine books, and other hard to find vaccine resources imported from around the world. We also offer nearly 200 books and videos on cutting-edge alternative health solutions, natural immunity, progressive parenting, natural childcare, AIDS, cancer, and more. Send for a FREE CATALOG: New Atlantean Press, PO Box 9638-925, Santa Fe, NM 87504. Or visit our internet *<u>Thinktwice Global Vaccine Institute</u>:* http://thinktwice.com

Neil Miller is a research journalist and natural health advocate.